Introduction to Oncogenes and
Molecular Cancer Medicine

Springer

New York
Berlin
Heidelberg
Barcelona
Budapest
Hong Kong
London
Milan
Paris
Singapore
Tokyo

Dennis W. Ross, M.D., Ph.D.
Department of Pathology
Forsyth Medical Center
Winston-Salem, NC 27103

Introduction to Oncogenes and Molecular Cancer Medicine

With 47 Illustrations

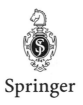

Springer

Dennis W. Ross, M.D., Ph.D.
Department of Pathology
Forsyth Medical Center
3333 Silas Creek Parkway
Winston-Salem, NC 27103
USA

Library of Congress Cataloging-in-Publication Data
Ross, D.W. (Dennis W.)
    Introduction to oncogenes and molecular cancer medicine / Dennis
  W. Ross
      p. cm.
    Includes bibliographical references and index.
    ISBN 0-387-98392-9 (softcover : alk. paper)
    1. Oncogenes.   2. Cancer—Molecular aspects.   I. Title.
    [DNLM: 1. Neoplasms—genetics.   2. Oncogenes.   3. Neoplasms—
  etiology.   4. Cell Transformation, Neoplastic.   QZ 202 R823i 1998]
  RC268.42.R67   1998
  616.99'4071—dc21
                                                              98-4703

Printed on acid-free paper.

Production managed by WordCrafters Editorial Services and supervised by Lesley Poliner; manufacturing supervised by Jacqui Ashri.
Typeset by MATRIX Publishing Services, York, PA.
Printed and bound by Maple-Vail Book Manufacturing Group, York, PA.
Printed in the United States of America.

9 8 7 6 5 4 3 2 1

ISBN 0-387-98392-9 Springer-Verlag New York Berlin Heidelberg   SPIN 10660234

This book
is dedicated to cancer patients
and to the renewed hope for the future
brought about by DNA technology.

Preface

The purpose of this book is to explore oncogenes and the current view of cancer as a molecular disease. I assume that you, the reader, have no specialized knowledge of molecular biology. Oncogenes are not a difficult subject, but they are new. Sometimes new ideas need to be considered several times from different points of view before they sink in. The basic principles of oncogenes and the molecular biology of cancer are explained first. Then clinical examples are used to demonstrate how our knowledge of the molecular basis of cancer improves diagnosis and treatment now, with promise for greater advances in the near future. The clinical examples in the second part of this book repeat and amplify the explanation of basic principles begun in the first part. Thus, Chapter 2 contains an explanation of how a dividing cell must pass through a checkpoint in the division cycle just before starting DNA synthesis. In Chapter 8, this concept is reexplored when we see how loss of tumor suppressor gene function in colon cancer removes this checkpoint. Mutated cells that should be stopped are allowed to divide; the result is a tumor. You may want to look at Table 11.1 right now. Ask yourself, "Do I understand the ideas and genetic mechanisms that are the basis for new molecular cancer therapies as listed in that table?" You will by the time you reach the end of this book!

Far from being all-inclusive, this book is a primer and hopefully a catalyst for your interest. My previous book, *Introduction to Molecular Medicine* (2nd ed. NY: Springer; 1996), covers other aspects of molecular biology applied to medicine, such as infectious and metabolic diseases. I also write a column, "Advances in the Science of Pathology," that appears in the *Archives of Pathology and Laboratory Medicine*. My writing and medical school teaching has convinced me that the best way to learn is to develop an interest and to have fun. Therefore the overriding style of this book is a travel guide where you and I are going on a short, fun, and adventurous trip.

As a guide, a glossary of key terms appears at the end of the book. These terms are printed in boldface when they first appear in the text. A short bibliography of pertinent references and suggested further reading appears at the end of each chapter. Some of these references are Web sites. Molecular biology lives on the Internet. It is a modern, fast-paced field in which young investigators type their newly discovered gene sequences into computer databases every night. Let's begin our trip.

Dennis W. Ross
Winston-Salem, North Carolina
June 1998

Acknowledgments

Marcel Bessis was my friend and teacher for many years. He taught me how to think critically and how to have fun in my work. I owe his memory the greatest debt. A number of people have reviewed draft chapters of this book and made helpful suggestions. I wish to thank them for their time and effort: Tom Grote, Judy Hopkins, Leonard Kaplow, Myla Lai-Goldman, Tehnaz Parakh, Mark Pettenati, Chuck Pippitt, Fredrick Reede, Jackie Smith, and Steve Schichman. My illustrator David Pounds has carefully endeavored to make my ideas more comprehensible through his artful drawings. Valerie Grooms has provided much valued secretarial help. I wish also to thank my partners in the Department of Pathology for making time available to me for this project, and my colleagues, the Medical Staff of Forsyth and Medical Park Hospitals, who have so encouraged me. I gratefully acknowledge grant support from The Blood Cell Fund.

Dennis W. Ross
Winston-Salem, North Carolina
June 1998

Contents

PART I

Basic Principles
of Molecular Biology

Molecular Biology of Cells

Overview

What Is a Gene?

*A **gene** is a piece of DNA* that encodes a packet of information that is part of a cell's permanent structure and is copied into daughter cells at division.*

The three essential elements of this definition are: DNA, information, and copied. Cancer is a disease that begins as a mutation in the DNA of a single cell. The abnormal bit of DNA distorts the information stored in a gene. In cancer, the misinformation relates to some error in the control of cell growth or senescence. The damaged gene is propagated to all the daughter cells when the DNA is copied. Because the error is propagated, cancer cells grow and become a disease. Fortunately most mutations in DNA do not result in cancer. Only when the mutated gene relates to cell growth, and only when the damage is such that it cannot be repaired, is cancer a possibility.

In this chapter we look into the molecular biology of the cell in order to understand in the following chapters how an alteration in DNA can result in cancer. We consider the richness of the entire human genome, its information content, and the physical structure of DNA. We then look in detail at the "anatomy" of a gene. The hereditary breast cancer susceptibility gene, BRCA1, serves as our first example. The principles of basic genetics as they relate to cancer, such as alleles and mutation, are reviewed.

---

*Genes can also be made of RNA as is the case in some viruses. In this book, I will usually stick to the major point of definition. However, sometimes the "minor" details are very important, particularly when they indicate an inconsistency that proves our knowledge is far from complete.

The Human Genome—Physical Structure

The DNA content of a single human cell is 7.1 picograms (10^{-12} grams). The DNA is present within the cell nucleus as a linear strand several meters long. This is a lot of "string" to pack into a sphere. A scaled-up model, making the cell nucleus the size of a basketball, would in turn scale the DNA to the thickness of a spider web strand 0.2 mm thick with an overall length of 200 kilometers. The packing of 200 kilometers of spider web into a basketball is difficult to imagine. The problem is even more complex when we include the requirement that we must be able to locate any one of the tens of thousands of genes strung out along that strand within fractions of a second (the time it takes for a cell to activate a gene). We also have to figure out a way to unwrap all 200 kilometers as the cell divides. Remember, we need to make two copies of the string and give one copy to each cell at division. For this task, we have 12 hours (the time it takes for a cell to copy its DNA). Figure 1.1 is a diagram of how packing of DNA occurs in a cell. The thread is looped two and a half times around small protein "bobbins" called histones. The histones themselves are grouped as a spiral collection that is in turn organized into loops and tufts, thousands of which make up the arms of a chromosome.

Table 1.1 gives some of the specific physical parameters of the human genome. There are 46 **chromosomes**, 22 pairs plus the sex chromosomes XX or XY. A cell is diploid, meaning it contains two copies of each chromosome and at least two copies of every gene. A male is a slight exception in that he has only one X chromosome, and only one copy of the genes located on X. The Y chromosome contains almost no genetic information. This is why males are subject to sex-linked inherited genetic diseases. If a man acquires from his mother a mutated copy of a gene on the X chromosome, there is no possibility of having another nonmutated correct copy on the other X chromosome.

The DNA molecule is the famous double helix inferred by Watson and Crick in 1953 from x-ray crystallography studies. Figure 1.2 shows the double helix of DNA. The double helix consists of ladder arms made up of deoxyribose. The rungs of the ladder are made up of pairs of two complementary bases. There are ten **base pairs (bp)** for every full twist of the helix. DNA uses only four bases as possible rungs, adenine (A), thymine (T), guanine (G), and cytosine (C). On the ladder rungs, A is always complemented (paired) with T, and G with C, for chemical reasons. The hydrogen bond between the base pairs is relatively weak. The DNA helix can be unzipped by separating the base pairs at this hydrogen bond. The two strands of the DNA helix need to unzip when the DNA is copied at cell division, or when

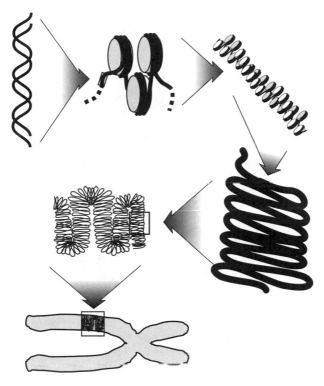

FIGURE 1.1. A schematic representation of the physical structure of DNA shows the multiple levels of packing into the final chromosome structure.

a portion of the strand is transcribed into RNA during gene expression. Each strand serves as the template for synthesizing a new complementary strand, as is shown in the lower half of Figure 1.2. The newly synthesized strand is complementary in the sense that everywhere there is an A on the original template, the complement reads T. G is complemented by C. When DNA

Table 1.1. Physical parameters of the human genome.

Number of base pairs = 6×10^9 (diploid genome)
Number of chromosomes = 22 pairs plus XX or XY
Length of DNA as a single linear strand $\sim$ 2 meters
Width of DNA double helix molecule = 2×10^{-9} meters
Helix rotates 360° every 10 bp = 3.4×10^{-9} meters
Weight of DNA in one cell = 7.1×10^{-12} grams
Number of genes = 100,000 (diploid genome)
Size of a gene = from 1000 bp to 200,000 bp; typical gene 30,000 bp

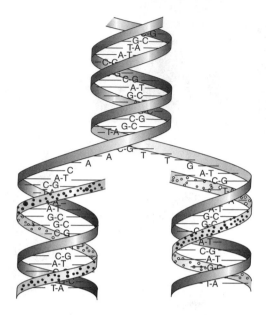

FIGURE 1.2. The DNA double helix consists of two complementary strands of paired bases. When the DNA is duplicated at cell division, or when DNA is transcribed into RNA, the double helix unwinds.

is copied incorrectly an error is introduced into the message, this is the start of cancer. To understand that key point as the start of cancer, we need to understand how information is stored in the gene.

The Human Genome—Information Content

The sequence of base pairs along a strand of the DNA helix spells out the message to the cell. The alphabet of the DNA language consists of the four letters, A,T,C, and G. The words are always three letters in length and are called codons. There are 64 possible **codons** in this language (four bases in three letter combinations, $4^3 = 64$). The words in this limited language are translated into amino acids, the building blocks of proteins. A gene's message specifies a protein. There is some redundancy in the genetic code. There are 64 codons that translate into only 20 amino acids used to make proteins. Several of the amino acids have up to four different codons. Three of the codons do not represent amino acids. They are the stop codons TAA, TAG, and TGA that serve as a "period" to terminate the message. The same genetic code translating DNA sequences to amino acids is used by every living organism so far discovered on the planet earth, from primitive bacteria and viruses to humans!

The entire human genome is 6 billion base pairs long. If spelled out and written as a book, the human genome would be the size of a medical school library. But the human genome does not contain essays or novels; it is a concise instruction manual specifying the structure of the proteins used to make up the cells of the human body. As we will see, a single misspelled "word" can cause cancer and other diseases. The information of the genome starts as base pairs (bp) read as three letter codons. The next level is the gene, typically 30,000 bp long. Within our library, a gene may be thought of as a book. A gene contains one complete message. There are about 100,000 genes in every human cell.

The human genome is a "read-only" library. The message is read by the cell, and copied at cell division, but new information is not written into the genome. Accidental errors are made in copying the genome; these errors are mutations. Mutations are usually harmless, and occasionally they cause disease such as cancer. All cancer results from mutation. Very rarely, a mutation produces a gene that makes the organism more adaptable to its environment. That animal and its progeny survive. This is the genetic basis of evolution, and this is the only way the human genome is rewritten. Evolution changes the message in our library only over a time span of tens of thousands of years.

I should say that the human genome *was* a "read-only" library. Genetic engineering now permits reading and writing into the genome. Some time this year or next, humans will have taken the tremendous and frightening step of writing artificially into our genome. Already genes have been introduced into human tissues to correct inherited disease. The first clinical human gene transplant was in 1991. An engineered copy of the *ADA* gene was introduced into bone marrow cells to correct hereditary immune deficiency. This was a somatic cell transplant affecting only one tissue. In many plants and animals, genetic engineering has been applied to the germ line cells. Once a new gene is introduced into the germ line, it persists in all future generations. These plants and animals are **transgenic,** meaning that their genetic component comes from means other than heredity. Transgenic plants and animals are created either to serve as models for human disease or to produce desirable special proteins. A transgenic cow, whose milk produces tissue plasminogen activator, is a dramatic example of the new industry of genetic engineering applied to pharmaceuticals. In DNA jargon, this process is called **pharming**. Genetic engineering on human embryos has not yet been undertaken for ethical reasons, but the technical capability exists. In Chapter 11 we will look in detail at human genetic engineering as a means of treating and preventing cancer.

Anatomy of a Gene

A gene is a blueprint for a protein. The base sequences in DNA are transcribed into RNA that is then translated into protein. Within the gene are also instructions that regulate its function, most specifically turning the gene on and off. To get right into the thick of it, let us consider a specific example of a cancer gene. The breast cancer susceptibility gene *BRCA*1 is complex and incompletely understood, but it is very important to clinical medicine. Our first look at this gene will raise a lot of issues. Some of these will remain unresolved until we have a second look at tumor suppressor genes in Chapter 4, and a more detailed look at the molecular genetics of breast cancer in Chapter 10. The normal physiologic function of *BRCA*1 is unknown. However, inherited mutations in this gene occur in about 1 in 800 women and are associated with a markedly increased risk of breast cancer. The lifetime risk of developing breast cancer in a person with an inherited mutation of *BRCA*1 is estimated at 60% to 85%.

We will look at the "anatomy" of the *BRCA*1 gene to get some idea of how big and complex the human genome is. Remember *BRCA*1 is one of 100,000 or so genes. Figure 1.3 is an example of what future textbooks of anatomy will look like. After medical students have struggled through gross and microscopic anatomy, they will be hit with a new level of detail, molecular anatomy. Understanding the structure of genes is necessary to using DNA technology for diagnosis and treatment. The left hand panel of Figure 1.3 is a schematic diagram of chromosome 17, showing the location of *BRCA*1. Specifically, *BRCA*1 is on the long arm of 17 (designated as q), within the second major light band distal to the centromere. Cytogenetic nomenclature denotes this location as 17q21. With a very good microscope and an optimal spread preparation of human chromosomes stained with Giemsa polychrome dye, something like the schematic of chromosome 17 shown in Figure 1.3 can actually be seen.

The middle panel of Figure 1.3 shows the genetic region around 17q21 with a few of the genes and mile posts established by the human genome project. D17S250 and D17S78 are survey marks from which we can measure our location as we move up and down the chromosome. *HER*2 and *RAR*a are genes. All of chromosome 17 represents about 200 million base pairs and 6000 genes. The middle panel of Figure 1.3 shows a region of about 1 to 2 million bp. The right hand panel is 100,000 bp. Progressing

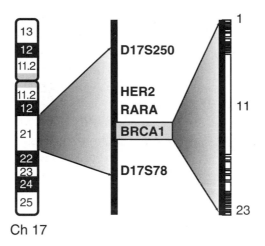

FIGURE 1.3. A gene map of *BRCA*1 begins by showing its location on the long arm of chromosome 17 at q2.1. The middle panel magnifies a 2-Mb span of this region encompassing several markers and genes adjacent to *BRCA*1. The right panel is a blow-up of the 23 exons of *BRCA*1 stretching over 100 Kb.

from left to right we have about 100x increased resolution in each panel. Genetic maps, like Figure 1.3, can be best viewed on the Internet. They are updated daily as frequent revisions and new discoveries are made. A good site at which to begin is www.ncbi.nlm.nih.gov. If you are interested in keeping up with the human genome project, you must use the Internet; that's where the action is. The human genome project progresses so rapidly and encompasses so much information, that of current technologies, only the Internet can cope (barely). The library analogy of the human genome that we considered earlier in this chapter actually lives on the Internet!

The right hand panel of Figure 1.3 shows a map of the *BRCA*1 gene. *BRCA*1 is a large gene, covering some 100,000 bp along the chromosome and consisting of 23 **exons**. An exon is a part of a gene consisting of base sequences that either regulate the gene's function or directly code for amino acids in the protein product of the gene. Spaces between exons are called **introns**. The introns are apparently nothing more than gaps with no known function. The genetic message is written with lots of gaps throughout the genome. In fact, only about 10% of the 6 billion bp in the human genome code for anything, the rest is "junk" DNA. For example, the whole of the Y chromosome in men is junk DNA. There is plenty of "blank paper" left for more messages in the human genome!

In the right hand panel of Figure 1.3, the exons are shown as rectangles whose length is proportional to the number of base pairs in each exon. The introns are shown only schematically as small gaps between the exons. Note that exon 11 in the middle of *BRCA1* is very large and accounts for about 60% of the gene. The first exon of *BRCA1* is an untranslated region or UTR, and presumably serves an as yet undiscovered control function. The other 22 exons code for the *BRCA1* protein.

The *BRCA1* gene is converted by the machinery of the cell into *BRCA1* protein. Figure 1.4 illustrates the steps of DNA to RNA to protein. Within the nucleus of the cell, an RNA transcript of the DNA copy of the gene is made. The entire 100,000-bp span of the gene is transcribed into RNA. Next, all of the sequences represented by the introns are spliced out. The dangling loops in the middle panel represent the portion of the RNA derived from intron sequences. These loops are spliced out and destroyed. This is 95% of the span of the gene that is thrown away! Only the RNA derived from the coding sequences of the exon remains. This final mRNA is much shorter than the 100,000-bp span of the gene as it spreads along the chromosome. The message has been spliced down to just the 5711-bp coding sequences. The mRNA sequences are next translated by the polyribosome machinery of the cell cytoplasm into a protein consisting

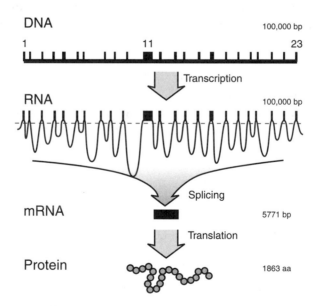

FIGURE 1.4. The *BRCA1* gene DNA sequences are made into a protein by the intermediate steps of: (1) transcription into RNA, (2) splicing into a much shorter mRNA, and (3) translation into protein.

of a chain of 1863 amino acids, as shown in the lower panel. The protein is a little shorter than we might calculate figuring on 3 bp to each amino acid ($5711/3 = 1903.67$). A few of the coding sequences in the mRNA start and stop the assembly of the protein and serve other housekeeping functions.

Over 200 mutations have so far been discovered in the *BRCA*1 gene in women with a hereditary predisposition to breast cancer. One of the first studied mutations was **185delAG**. We will consider this mutation in detail right now, to get a feel of how mutations mess things up. Later in this chapter, and then repeatedly throughout this book, we will be discussing different types of mutations and how they cause cancer.

In the 185delAG mutation, the bases adenine (A) and guanine (G) at positions 185 and 186 are erroneously deleted. Think of what will result from this mutation. . . . With the loss of two bases from the coding sequence near the start of the gene, the entire remainder of the message will be read out of sequence. The polyribosomes read three bases at a time as a codon. If two are dropped out, there will be a **frame shift** in the reading of the message. Every amino acid following this deletion will be incorrect and the resulting protein coded for by the mutant *BRCA*1 gene will be defective.

Figure 1.5 is a listing of the DNA sequences from bases 180 to 248 for the *BRCA*1 gene. The upper panel of Figure 1.5 shows the correct DNA sequence as capital letters beginning with the codon ATC. Underneath the DNA sequence is the translation of each codon into its corresponding amino acid written as a lower case three letter abbreviation. The codon ATC translates into isoleucine (ile). The bases at 185 and 186 are highlighted in the upper panel. The lower panel shows what happens in 185delAG with the loss of these two bases. The amino acid translation downstream of the mutation is incorrect because the codons are not being read in the proper phase. This is a frame shift mutation and occurs whenever one or two bases are deleted. In this shifted reading frame, the *BRCA*1 protein is assembled with an incorrect sequence of amino acids. Furthermore, the frame shifted message reaches a premature termination of the protein long before the natural end at 1863 amino acids. The frame shift has produced mRNA that is more or less a random sequence of codons. In this "nonsense" message a stop codon is randomly generated. Recall that 3 out of the 64 possible codons are periods that stop translation. **Nonsense** messages generated by frame shift mutations terminate quickly when they reach a randomly generated stop codon. The mutated sequence shown in the lower panel of Figure 1.5 ends when the codon TGA is translated into a stop.

Only correct gene sequences have long **open reading frames**. In the

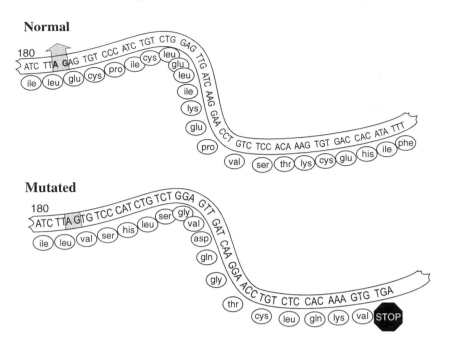

FIGURE 1.5. The genomic sequences for bases 180 to 248 of *BRCA*1 for both the normal and a mutated form are shown. The del185AG mutation causes a frame shift that results in the early termination of the protein with a stop codon, TGA.

human genome project, one of the first ways a new gene is recognized is as an open reading frame. Automated sequencing of DNA generates data as a string of A, T, G, and Cs. A computer scans the data and notes whenever a long open reading frame is detected, indicating a gene. Stretches of DNA that do not have a long open reading frame are "junk" spacing between genes. Remember that about 90% of the genome is this junk spacing. The computer must try to read the sequence data in all three of the possible reading frames. Only the correct frame within a gene will be open, that is, have a long stretch of DNA code with no stop codons.

As an optional exercise try to prove this to yourself. Use the sequence data for *BRCA*1 in the top panel of Figure 1.5. I have already shown you that the open reading frame begins at position 180 with the codon ATC. Try the other two possible reading frames beginning with position 181, first codon TCT; and beginning with position 182, first codon CTT. Mark out groups of three bases (a codon) for these two alternate reading frames in Figure 1.5. See how far you can go before you reach one of the STOP codons, TAA, TAG, or TGA. Have you convinced yourself that only the correct reading frame remains open? (Thanks for marking up the book. Now other people will know that you have read it, and they will go buy their own copy.)

The 185delAG mutation is only one of the 200 or so mutations that have been discovered in the families of women with a hereditary disposition to breast cancer. This particular mutation is much more common in Jewish women of Eastern European descent, where the incidence is approximately 1 in 100. An important feature of genetic traits is that they are not evenly distributed throughout the population, but concentrated within specific ethnic groups. Consider the complexities this brings to the problem of genetic testing. Which mutation should be looked at in which patients? We will return to the specific problem of genetic testing for *BRCA*1 in Chapter 10. There we will see how advanced DNA technology combined with medical judgment offers a reasonable solution. To find mutations in *BRCA*1, we can use either direct sequencing of DNA, or look for premature termination of the *BRCA*1 protein.

Basic Genetics

We have already realized that the human genome is diploid, with two copies of every chromosome. However, the chromosomes are not necessarily identical. Each gene has a specific location on a chromosome, but there are multiple alternative forms of a gene, called **alleles**. Consider the gene for the beta chain of hemoglobin located on chromosome 11. There are many alleles (multiple alternative forms) of this gene. In fact, hundreds of variations of the normal hemoglobin chain genes are known. One diploid human will possess two alleles of the beta chain gene, one on each of the two chromosomes 11. Many of the allelic variations of the beta chain gene produce no disease or detectable abnormality. Some, like the sickle cell allele, produce a laboratory abnormality (in vitro sickling) when present as one copy, and a clinical disease when present as two copies. The sickle cell gene (an allelic variation of the hemoglobin beta chain) is **recessive**. This means that if only one copy of the abnormality is present, disease is not apparent since the remaining normal beta globin allele is capable of producing sufficient functional protein. If only one allele present is sufficient to cause an abnormality, the allele is said to be **dominant.**

In cancer genetics, the situation is rarely as straightforward as simple dominant or recessive alleles. Cancer is caused by mutation in control genes, the effects of which are somewhat remote. In the mutation del185AG of *BRCA*1, one allele is mutated and the other is normal.

Nevertheless, a woman with this mutation will likely develop breast cancer some 40 years after birth. The normal *BRCA*1 protein produced by the nonmutated allele on the other chromosome 17 must somehow become disrupted. In Chapter 4 we will discuss the mechanism called loss of heterozygosity by which this comes about.

Mutations come in many sizes and kinds (see Table 1.2). A mutation can be as simple as a single base switch. The sickle cell mutation is a switch of an A for a T at the twentieth position in the beta globin gene. This results in the change of one codon and causes a corresponding switch in one amino acid. Glutamine (glu) replaces valine (val) as the sixth amino acid in the protein encoded by the gene. Another example of a point mutation occurs in the H-*ras* oncogene. Single base substitutions at codons 12, 59, or 61 result in a marked increase in the cell transforming ability of the H-*ras* protein (as will be discussed in Chapter 3). These *ras* point mutations are commonly seen as acquired mutations in colon, pancreas, and lung tumors. Besides a simple switch of one base for another, deletions of bases are a common type of mutation. These produce frame shifts in the reading of the codons as we saw for del185AG *BRCA*1. Mutations can also occur as a loss of much larger portions of DNA, up to hundreds of thousands of base pairs. The tumor suppressor gene p53 is frequently mutated due to loss of relatively long segments of the gene. The **p53** gene presents as an acquired somatic mutation in up to 50% of cancers. An additional mechanism for mutation is switching pieces of the genome out of their normal places as occurs in a **chromosomal translocation**. An example of this is the chromosomal translocation of the c-*myc* oncogene from its normal location on chromosome 8 into the immunoglobulin gene on chromosome 14, resulting in Burkitt's lymphoma (as will be discussed in Chapters 3 and 7). Many mutations result in an abnormal protein that causes abnormal or loss of function. Some mutations occur in the nonencoding portion of a gene. In these instances, the protein coming from the gene is not abnormal, but it is not produced at the right time or in the

Table 1.2. Types of DNA mutations.

Name	Example
Point mutation	Codon 12, 59, or 61 in H-*ras* oncogene; colon, pancreas, and lung cancer
Frame shift deletion	del185AG in *BRCA*1 tumor suppressor gene; breast cancer
Chromosomal translocation	Translocation of c-*myc* oncogene from chromosome 8 into immunoglobulin gene on chromosome 14; Burkitt's lymphoma

right amounts. Table 1.2 summarizes these various types of gene mutations with examples relevant to cancer.

Not every alteration in DNA produces an abnormality, in fact most do not. If a change in DNA occurs between genes, generally no effect occurs. Such a change is called a **polymorphism**. A difficult distinction related to the definition of a mutation is whether a given change is an abnormality or just different. Some people use the word mutation only for a deleterious change in a gene, and call all other changes a polymorphism. I, for example, am bald. Is this an acceptable variation on normal hair-bearing, or an abnormality? Whatever your answer, I must tell you that almost all geneticists would respond that I carry the mutant gene for male pattern baldness.

A very important distinction for us to make is the difference between an acquired **somatic** cell mutation and an inherited **germ line** mutation. Classical genetics deals mostly with inherited traits due to genes present in the germ line received from two parents. The molecular biology of cancer deals mostly with acquired somatic mutations that were not present at birth. Somatic mutations begin in a single cell as the result of an error in DNA copying and repair. Only a few cancers are related to an inherited germ line mutation. The example of *BRCA1* and inherited breast cancer susceptibility that we have used in this chapter, accounts for only 5% of breast tumors. Even in this instance, further somatic mutations must occur for a tumor to develop.

Summary

In this first chapter, we have laid out the basics of DNA, molecular biology, and genetics. The physical size and characteristics of the human genome have been dissected and reconstructed, blown up to 200 kilometers of spider web in a basketball. The vast information of the genome has been compared to a library, with each gene a separate book. We have looked at the map of one gene, BRCA1 on chromosome 17, as a string of 23 exons spread out over 100,000 bases. Yet we have seen that the deletion of only two bases at position 185 and 186 results in a near certainty of breast cancer. The cell loses its reading frame in translating the protein. We find that mutations come in every size from a single misspelled word up to switching large pieces of chromosomes, equivalent to scrambling a whole floor of our imaginary library.

The next step in our understanding of the molecular biology of cancer will be to trace how errors in DNA result in altered cell growth. In the next chapter, we move from the behavior of molecules up to that of cells. Bad DNA becomes uncontrolled cell growth.

References

Alberts B, Bray D, Lewis J, Raff M, Roberts K, Watson J, eds. *Molecular Biology of the Cell*, 3rd ed. New York: Garland Publications; 1994.

Genomic and Genetic Resources on the World Wide Web: http://www.nhgri.nih.gov

Lodish H, Baltimore D, Berk A, Zipursky SL, Matsudaira P, Darnell J, eds. *Molecular Cell Biology*. 3rd ed. New York: Scientific American Books; 1995.

Lewin B. *Genes VI*. Oxford: Oxford Univ Press; 1997.

Ross DW. *Introduction to Molecular Medicine*. 2nd ed. New York: Springer-Verlag; 1996.

Cell Growth and Senescence

Overview

A living human cell is both a single entity and part of a multicellular organism. Cancer is a disease of uncontrolled cell growth, where a cell with mutated DNA stops following the normal instructions that govern its life as part of the organism. A cancer cell is a rebel. The fall from normal law abiding cooperation to self-perpetuating out-of-control rebellion is not a single step. Cancer cells may be only slightly deranged, paralleling the functions of their normal counterparts. This results in a slow growing, well differentiated tumor. However, with each successive cell division, cancer cells lose more of their control. The cancer progressively becomes a fast growing dedifferentiated tumor where the malignant cells are guided only by primitive internal instructions that speed their replication.

The cell division cycle, with its DNA replication and repair phases, checkpoints, and programmed cell death, is how cells are controlled. The cell division cycle permits the body's renewal and remodeling of tissues. Cancer is fundamentally a derangement of this process. We will study the normal cell division cycle in some detail, while looking at the steps where cancer cells depart from the normal program. This basic science is central to our knowledge of cancer as a cellular and molecular disease.

Cell Culture Model

A model of the cell division cycle much used in research is **in vitro** cell culture. If a sample of human tissue, typically skin fibroblasts, is disaggregated into a single cell suspension and then placed in a nutrient medium, the cells will grow. The necessary environment for cell growth in addition to the complex nutrient medium includes hormone-like growth factors, a plastic surface for cell attachment, and a 37°C incubator with a 5% carbon dioxide atmosphere. Under these conditions, the skin fibroblasts will grow continuously. Each cell will divide every 24 hours into two new daughter cells. There will be very little cell death. Only about one cell in ten will fail after the culture becomes established. In about two months, after approximately 50 cell divisions, the cells will stop dividing, become senescent, and then die. This is "normal" behavior for human cells taken out of the body and placed in this in vitro culture.

A number of factors including certain viruses, chemical carcinogens, and radiation can **transform** the cells so that they divide continuously. The cell culture no longer dies out after two months, but continues indefinitely. The cells are said to be transformed or immortalized. This is an in vitro model of **neoplastic** cell growth. The normal molecular events that control cell division and the eventual programmed cell death are pretty well understood. The changes that occur in transformed cells tell us a lot about cancer.

Cell Cycle

The cell division cycle is best explained as a diagram showing the interrelationships of a number of events as shown in Figure 2.1. The circle in the right half of the figure is the traditional representation for continuously dividing cells. This part of the cycle consists of **G1** (gap one), followed by **S** (a phase of DNA synthesis), followed by **G2** (gap two), and ending with **M** (mitosis). It's what we discovered first. The left half of the diagram shows the more recently discovered quiescent phases and checkpoints in the cycle. **G0** is a reservoir for quiescent cells to leave the actively dividing portion of the cycle. G0 cells can, under the appropriate stimulus, reenter the active cycle at G1. Quiescent cells in G0, when they have completed their functional usefulness, receive a signal that causes them to undergo **apoptosis** (also called programmed cell death). Actively dividing cells go through a **checkpoint** at the G1/S boundary. If there is DNA damage that cannot be repaired, the cell will not pass the checkpoint and instead will receive the instruction to undergo apoptosis. A second less well understood checkpoint occurs at the G2/M boundary. The genes that regulate the cell cycle with its checkpoints, DNA repair, and apoptosis are oncogenes and tumor suppressor genes. This is where the control of cell proliferation occurs; this is where an error leads to cancer. Chapters 3 and 4 will look in more detail at specific oncogenes and

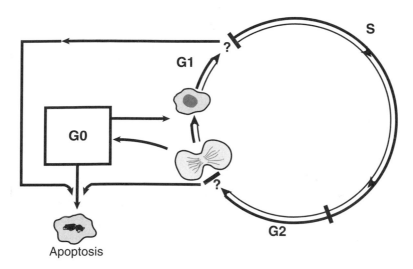

FIGURE 2.1. The cell division cycle is defined by the major events that control proliferation. Actively dividing cells progress from G1, to DNA synthesis (S), to G2, then to mitosis (M). At several checkpoints (?), the cell's progress is tested and if damage is detected the cell dies (apoptosis). G0 is a reservoir of quiescent, nondividing cells.

tumor suppressor genes. Our goal for the moment is to achieve an overview of normal cell proliferation and how it can go awry.

The balance between increase in cell number by mitosis and loss of cell number by apoptosis is how a tissue maintains itself. When more cells are needed, the balance shifts toward mitosis. When fewer cells are needed, the balance shifts toward apoptosis. For some tissues, like the skin, cell turnover is very high. Cells at the base of the epidermis are actively dividing. Cells above the basal layer are quiescent from the point of view of cell division. They, however, are active in their functional role and continue to synthesize keratin. These cells are in G0. The mature squamous cells near the surface of the epidermis undergo apoptosis, die, and slough off the skin when their functional role is over.

Figure 2.2 gives results of an experiment that looks in more detail at cells growing in the actively dividing portion of the cell cycle. These data are from my first published experiment (Sinclair and Ross, 1969); and as such I have a natural but unwarranted attachment to this figure. Affection for my own experiment is understandable to anyone who has spent time in the lab. Research is the slowest and least certain way to answer a question. Looking the answer up in a book, asking some supposed expert, or simply speculating on what the answer should be are all much faster than

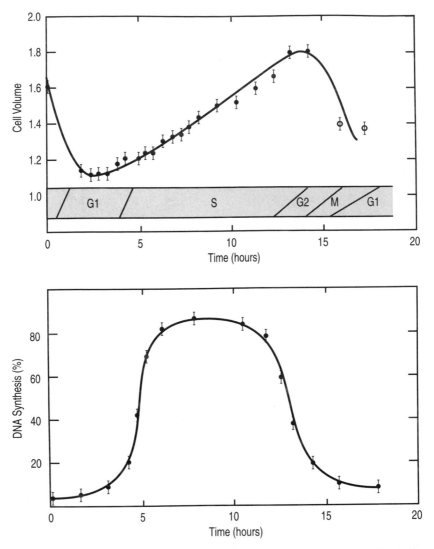

FIGURE 2.2. Cell growth and DNA synthesis during the cycle. A cell culture is synchronized, starting with mitotic cells at 0 hours. The progress of the cell cycle is measured by cell volume and percent cells synthesizing DNA, determined at half-hour intervals. These data determine the length of M, G1, S, and G2 compartments of the cell cycle.

the experimental method. Nevertheless, finding the answer in the lab, besides being satisfying, gives deep insight into just how good or complete that answer is. In this experiment the cell culture was synchronized, meaning that at time t = 0, all the cells had just completed mitosis. Over the next division cycle, cell volume and the presence of DNA synthesis were measured at half-hour intervals. These cells were a transformed culture of Chinese hamster fibroblasts. Back in the 1960s when I did this experiment, it was much easier to grow Chinese or Syrian hamster cells than human cells. At that time, we did not understand the growth factors needed by human cells. Hamster cells also kept their chromosomes in good order when cultured, whereas most other animal or human cell cultures did not (for unknown reasons). These cells completed the division cycle in about 17 hours, somewhat faster than the typical 24 hours for human fibroblasts.

In Figure 2.2, we can see how the phases of the cell cycle are determined. At 0 hours, the newly divided cells are all growing in volume, but they are not synthesizing DNA. The cell growth continues smoothly throughout the whole cycle. DNA synthesis on the other hand is discontinuous, beginning abruptly at 5 hours and ending at 12 hours. The mid portion of the cycle was named S phase and the gaps before and after DNA synthesis, G1 and G2, respectively.

DNA Synthesis

Within the 12 or so hours of S phase, a cell must double its DNA in order to have two copies to partition between the two daughter cells at mitosis. A number of complex enzyme driven events occur during DNA synthesis. The DNA must be unraveled, and finally the double helix itself unzipped. **Replicons** (points of DNA copying) spring up throughout the genome. The replicons copy DNA from each of the two strands of the double helix at a rate of several thousand base pairs per second. We have a total of 6 billion base pairs to copy, so hundreds or thousands of replicons must be working simultaneously to get the job done in half a day. During all of this, the cell must also maintain normal functions requiring gene expression with transcription of DNA into RNA and translation into proteins.

Many of the chemotherapy drugs that we employ in the treatment of cancer take advantage of the special requirements of cells undergoing DNA synthesis. These drugs are most effective in rapidly dividing tumors. The measurement of the fraction of cells undergoing DNA synthesis by flow cytometry is relatively easy (see also Chapter 6). A fluorescent dye that binds to DNA is added to a disaggregated suspension of tumor cells. The sample is passed as a narrow stream, one cell at a time, through a laser. The amount of fluorescence is measured and is converted into a cell-by-cell measurement of DNA content. Cells in G1 have a normal component of two copies of each chromosome plus the sex chromosomes. This is about 7 picograms of DNA per cell, and is defined as

diploid DNA. Half normal, or **haploid**, DNA only occurs in germ cells such as the sperm and oocyte. Cells in G2 and M have twice the normal amount of DNA and are **tetraploid**. Any cell with a DNA content between diploid and tetraploid is in the process of doubling its DNA and is calculated as being in S phase. The **S phase fraction** of a tumor is both a useful prognostic parameter as well as a guide to choice of chemotherapy. Some tumors have markedly abnormal chromosome karyotypes due to accumulated mutations. Their DNA content is **aneuploid**. Aneuploid means not normal ploidy. Calculation of S phase fraction in aneuploid tumors is more complex, but possible.

DNA Repair

During the copying of 6 billion base pairs in the S phase of the cell division cycle, a number of errors will be made. Our best estimate is that about 600,000, or 0.01% of the base pairs will have been copied incorrectly during the first pass of DNA synthesis. The DNA synthesis mechanism is very, very good but not perfect. These errors will be for the most part corrected. If they cannot be corrected, the cell will in all likelihood be destroyed later at a checkpoint. There are a number of different DNA repair mechanisms operating within the cell nucleus. Before the cell cycle is complete, due to DNA repair the error rate is down from 10^{-4} to approximately 10^{-9}. That means that out of 6 billion base pairs, one will have been replicated incorrectly!

DNA repair works not only in correcting copy errors, but also to correct other damage to DNA that occurs in nondividing cells. Table 2.1 lists the known important types of repair. Recall our primary thesis of this book. Cancer results from an error in DNA that causes unregulated cell growth. Therefore we are very interested in (1) mutations that cause DNA errors, and (2) failures of the DNA repair system that allow these errors to go uncorrected.

Table 2.1. DNA repair mechanisms.

Type	Mechanism
Direct repair	Replaces a single alkylated base
Excision repair	Removes and replaces short "distorted" sequences, such as DNA adducts
Mismatch base repair	Repair of sequences with noncomplementary bases
Postreplication repair	Damaged DNA not copied during S, gap later filled
Cell cycle checkpoint	DNA damage detected, delay before progression in cell cycle

Checkpoints

The staging of events during the cell division cycle is controlled by a group of enzymes called cyclin-dependent kinases (Cdk) that interact with other proteins called cyclins. At the G1/S boundary a necessary level of cyclin E/Cdk2 complex is required to allow for the cell to pass on into S phase (active DNA synthesis). The p53 tumor suppressor gene can slow or block progression through this checkpoint by inhibiting the formation of these complexes. The normal function of p53 is to slow down the cell cycle when DNA damage is detected. This gives the cell a chance to repair the DNA before it replicates its DNA. Another cyclin/Cdk complex appears to modulate the G2/M checkpoint. Again this gives the cell a chance to repair damage, such as DNA strand breaks, before undergoing mitosis.

A number of the hereditary syndromes exist in which DNA repair is defective. Some examples are given in Table 2.2. Patients with these syndromes either cannot repair DNA damage or they do not have checkpoint controls. That is, they do not have time to repair damage. Patients with Xeroderma pigmentosum have decreased repair of ultraviolet radiation induced DNA strand breaks. They have a marked increase in skin cancers as a result. Patients with familial ataxia telangiectasia have near normal DNA repair capabilities. Their cells however, do not delay at the checkpoints when DNA damage occurs. In response to irradiation, or other DNA damage, their cells progress to S phase and mitosis before repairs are completed. This leads to the marked increase in cancer incidence in ataxia telangiectasia patients.

The familial syndromes listed in Table 2.2 are quite rare. These patients account for only a very small fraction of cancers. These syndromes do demonstrate the importance of DNA repair as a means of preventing cancer. In Chapter 4, we shall discuss acquired (as opposed to hereditary)

Table 2.2. Examples of inherited syndromes with defective DNA repair.

Syndrome	Mechanism
Ataxia telangiectasia	Failure of G1/M checkpoint delay
Bloom's syndrome	Fragile chromosomes
Fanconi's anemia	Defect in repair of DNA cross-links
Hereditary nonpolyposis colorectal cancer	hMSH2, defect in mismatch repair
Li–Fraumeni syndrome	Inherited p53 defect, failure after second mutation
Xeroderma pigmentosum	Defect in excision repair of UV induced DNA pyrimidine dimers

damage to cancer repair mechanisms due to mutation in tumor suppressor genes. In most cancers, the defect in DNA repair occurs as a somatic cell mutation rather than an inherited defect.

Apoptosis

The major role of apoptosis, or programmed cell death, as a means of deleting cells to control growth and development of tissues, has only recently come to be appreciated. The counterpart of apoptosis, mitosis or cell birth, has been appreciated for centuries. The lack of appreciation of apoptosis probably relates to its inclusion, erroneously, as a form of necrosis. Necrosis is tissue death from any form usually secondary to an insult. Apoptosis is supposed to happen in cells. Apoptosis happens rapidly, in about 30 minutes. The cell dies by DNA fragmentation, nuclear chromatin condensation, and the formation of cytoplasmic buds.

A cell undergoing apoptosis can be recognized under the microscope by a number of morphologic features that distinguish apoptosis from other forms of cell death. Apoptosis involves single isolated cells rather than a confluent portion of a tissue. In apoptosis, the cell nucleus and cytoplasm condense. The cytoplasm then buds and forms apoptotic bodies containing cell organelles. Phagocytic cells engulf these bodies and their contents are degraded by fusion within lysosomes. An inflammatory response is not produced in apoptosis, in distinction to necrosis where inflammation is an important accompanying factor. Biochemical events occur in parallel with theses morphologic changes. The most important is the condensation of nuclear chromatin and the rapid degradation of nuclear DNA by cleavage between nucleosomes. The degraded DNA demonstrates a ladder of oligonucleotide fragments of 180 to 200 bp as seen on an electrophoretic gel, characteristic of apoptosis. The rapid destruction of DNA in apoptosis may occur to prevent a dying cell from passing on intact DNA fragments to its neighbors.

The mechanisms by which apoptosis are regulated to form part of the homeostatic processes that control tissue growth and development are known only in part. Several genes are known to modulate or initiate apoptosis, probably as part of multiple alternate pathways. The growth control oncogene c-*myc* can act to stimulate either mitosis or apoptosis depending on the level of c-*myc* protein expressed and other costimuli. The tumor suppressor gene p53 "uses" apoptosis as a final step in DNA repair and protection from mutations. When a cell's DNA is damaged, p53 protein causes a prolongation of the G1 phase of the cell division cycle. The cell is paused at the G1/S checkpoint. If the DNA cannot be repaired during the pause, then p53 causes apoptosis to occur and the cell suicides rather than propagate possible mutations. Deletion of p53 function is very common in a wide range of tumors demonstrating the importance of this protective mechanism. The *bcl*-2 oncogene has the opposite effect of p53 in tumors. Rather than promoting apoptosis, *bcl*-2 blocks it. The role of *bcl*-2 has been best studied in lymphoid malignancies where a translocation of *bcl*-2 from chromosome 18 to the immunoglobulin locus on chromosome 14 causes increased expression of *bcl*-2. A malignant clone of lymphocytes bearing t(14;18) usually has only a low proliferative fraction, but the clone grows because it has near zero programmed cell death (see also Chapter 7).

The number of cells in a tissue undergoing apoptosis can be measured using flow cytometry or other biochemical methods. For some tumors, an apoptotic index may be a more useful clinical parameter than the S phase fraction measure of proliferation. Apoptosis in tumors increases following irradiation and immune therapies. Measuring apoptosis in vivo or in vitro following treatment may predict the effectiveness of the therapy.

Aging—An Aside

At the start of this chapter we saw that in our tissue culture model, neoplastic cells were immortalized. That is, cancer cells do not "age." They are capable of an unlimited number of cell divisions. This raises the question, "What is aging?" Although aging of an organism is not the same as aging in a cell, it is worth discussing as an aside in our attempt to understand, "What is cancer?"

Aging is the decreased repair of damage to tissues and loss of function that occurs over an organism's natural lifespan. Aging is dramatically species specific. The "natural" maximal lifespan of a human being is about 120 years; 40 for a chimpanzee; 30 for a dog; and only 3 for the laboratory white mouse, yet all age similarly. A human infant and a puppy may start life together, but by the time the child is a teenager, the dog will be old with stiff joints and sagging, wrinkled skin. What mechanisms control aging and the timing of its onset?

Most recent theories of aging center around the accumulation of cellular and molecular damage. In the cell culture model, nonneoplastic human fibroblasts have a limited division potential in vitro. Cells from older people will undergo fewer divisions than those from children. After a certain number of divisions, all cells eventually become senescent in the G1 phase of the cell cycle. Fusion of a senescent cell with a young cell in-

hibits division of the young cell. Addition of mRNA extracted from senescent cells has the same effect. This senescence of fibroblasts results from gene products (such as p21 and p53 associated WAF1, to be specific) that inhibit DNA synthesis and thus block cell division. Thus cellular senescence is the result of genetically controlled processes that irreversibly inhibit DNA synthesis. But what is the initiating factor?

*Multiple pathways appear to trigger cellular senescence. One such pathway is telomere shortening. **Telomeres** are genetic elements located at the distal end of chromosomes. Telomeres consist of about 15,000 bp of repetitive DNA sequences. The six bases TTAGGG are repeated thousands of times. They are replicated by a special DNA **telomerase**. However, at each division, a small piece of the telomere, about 100 bp, is not copied. Thus, telomeres become shortened over progressive cell divisions. At some point, this shortening induces inhibition of DNA synthesis and senescence. Cancer cells, as we will discuss in Chapter 5, rebuild the cleaved piece from the telomere at each division. Cancer cells do not age as measured by their telomeres.*

Another pathway to cellular senescence is accumulation of unrepaired DNA damage. DNA diffusely degrades over time. Most damage to DNA is repaired as we have shown, but some persists. For example, as the organism ages, more DNA is methylated. This inhibits the correct transcription of DNA to RNA, and leads to mutation when the DNA is replicated during division. DNA adducts are another example of potentially permanent damage. Adducts are formed when certain compounds bind tightly to DNA. These compounds are by definition mutagenic, since like methylation, they alter the function and copying of DNA. (This will also be discussed in Chapter 5, the section on carcinogenesis). Unrepaired damage to DNA, whether due to radiation, mutagenic chemicals, or degradation, increases over an organism's lifespan. After a certain point, accumulated damage causes an inhibition of DNA synthesis similar to that seen in senescent fibroblasts. Why should such damage reach a critical level after only one to two years in a mouse, while taking decades for the same effect to occur in humans?

Some overall clock must be involved in controlling the rate and timing of aging. Several "clock" genes have been found in the nematode that can, when manipulated, greatly alter the lifespan of that simple worm. In humans, this clock, if it exists, has not been found. Some alternate, noncellular theories of aging in humans propose that the neuroendocrine system is our master time clock. Others have proposed that the immune system or the central nervous system controls aging.

Two diseases characterized by premature human aging confirm what we know so far about cellular senescence. The gene that causes Werner's syndrome, one form of hereditary premature aging with diminished in vitro fibroblast doublings, has recently been cloned. Werner's syndrome patients apparently have a defective DNA helicase (one of the enzymes necessary for replication and repair). This would be expected to lead to a more rapid accumulation of incorrectly repaired double-strand DNA breaks. Patients with progeria, an even more rapid premature aging, start life with shortened telomeres. Thus they reach the critical "too short" limit much sooner than normal subjects.

A final and critical issue in the biology of aging is to recognize the difference between diseases associated with advancing age such as cancer, atherosclerosis, or dementia; and aging itself. There is significant disagreement as to what is aging and what is disease in older humans. Aging is probably best viewed currently as the result of many factors both internal (genetically programmed) and external (damage to tissues) that combine to impede progressively the function of the entire organism.

Summary

In this second chapter, we have seen how the growth of cells is regulated. The cell division cycle meters the flow of cells towards either replication or senescence. Damaged cells are repaired or committed to programmed destruction via apoptosis. The repair of damage to DNA is affected by many different mechanisms, culminating in cell cycle checkpoints that pass, delay, or reject the cell. The rare inherited syndromes with defective DNA repair all have a very high cancer incidence. Cancer is the final outcome of unrepaired DNA. The aging of cells and of the body is an additional facet of the regulation of cell growth. Cancer cells do not age as measured by telomere shortening and ability to divide continuously in cell culture. The controls of cell growth are numerous. Breakdown in any one of the multiple control and repair mechanisms is one step in multistage carcinogenesis. In the next chapters, we will examine in detail the genes responsible for control of cell growth; in Chapter 3, the oncogenes and in Chapter 4, the tumor suppressor genes.

References

Hartwell LH, Kastan MB. Cell cycle control and cancer. *Science*. 1994;266: 1821–1828.

Hetts SW. To die or not to die. An overview of apoptosis and its role in disease. *JAMA* 1998;279:300–307.

Kaufmann WK, Paules RS. DNA damage and cell cycle checkpoints. *FASEB J*. 1996;10:238–247.

Ross, DW. Biology of aging. *Arch Pathol Lab Med*. 1996;120:1148.

Ross, DW. Apoptosis. *Arch Pathol Lab Med*. 1997;121:83.

Sinclair WK, Ross DW. Modes of growth in mammalian cells. *Biophys. J*. 1969;9:1056–1070.

Smith JR, Pereira-Smith OM. Replicative senescence: Implications for in vivo aging and tumor suppression. *Science*. 1996;273:63–66.

Oncogenes: Control of
Cell Growth and Senescence

Overview

An oncogene is a growth control gene that when mutated "causes" a normal cell to become neoplastic.* In Chapters 1 and 2, we explored basic molecular and cellular biology. A few examples demonstrated how loss of control might lead to unregulated cell proliferation. Now we are ready to get into the molecular biology of cancer at a deeper level. The cell signal pathway is the connection between the DNA in the cell nucleus and regulatory signals from the outside. Most proteins that make up the links in this path are the products of oncogenes. When a cancer cell stops obeying the regulatory signals that make cells function as part of the body, it is due to a mutation in an oncogene. Oncogenes are the central feature in the molecular basis of cancer.

Analogy: The Registrar's Mutation

Let's begin this chapter with an analogy that demonstrates how an oncogene mutation can cause a neoplasm. Consider a medical school library. There are many books, containing about as much information as is present in the human genome. A few of these books deal with the organizational structure of the medical school. In one of them, *Instructions for Enrollment, Course Registration, and Graduation,* there is a mutation. Near the end of the book, the text has been erroneously modified by a translo-

---

*By Chapter 5, I hope to establish clearly that cancer is a multistep process. No one event can be said to be the cause of cancer. However, the mutation of an oncogene is a signature event.

cation of a paragraph from near the beginning. In the original correct version, the fourth year medical student is instructed to take his or her grade transcript to the registrar in exchange for a diploma. In the mutated version, immediately following "take your transcript to the registrar," the words "and receive your first year course assignments" have been inserted. The correct instruction "and exchange for a diploma" have been overwritten by a translocation from the instructions for entering students. What is the result of this mutation in the "Instructions" book for medical students? Fourth year students, instead of leaving and progressing to their mature function as physicians, return to the intermediate function of first year students. Within a few years, the classrooms are overcrowded inside the medical school, while outside there is a shortage of physicians. Let us compare this analogy to the molecular basis of a form of leukemia.

Acute promyelocytic leukemia is associated with a chromosome translocation t(15;17) that moves the retinoic acid receptor gene (*RAR*a) from chromosome 15 to 17, inserting it next to a gene called *PML*. The result is a neoplastic leukemic cell that has arrested maturation. The leukemic promyelocytes pack the marrow, whereas the peripheral blood becomes depleted of mature neutrophils. The cause is a translocation of a growth control gene that makes the cell unresponsive to growth factors. Acute promyelocytic leukemia can be treated with high doses of retinoic acid (vitamin A) that override the growth factor insensitivity and force maturation. The treatment is not usually a permanent cure because genetic instability in the leukemic cells leads to further mutations.

Many, many mutations are possible in the human genome. A mutation in an oncogene leads to cancer because the instructions controlling cell division have been damaged. There are hundreds of known oncogenes and so many possible ways to go wrong. After reading this chapter we may wonder why cancer does not occur more frequently! That despair will be tempered in Chapter 4 where we will consider tumor suppressor genes whose normal function is to prevent tumor cells from propagating. Tumor suppressor genes work "down stream" of oncogenes. They provide a means to stop a mutated cell from propagating. In Chapter 5, we will draw both oncogenes and tumor suppressor genes into a unified theory of the molecular basis of cancer.

Historic Background

Some confusion about "what is an oncogene?" derives from scientists' previous incomplete understanding. It is worthwhile as an antidote to this confusion to consider how, within a relatively short time, our definition of an oncogene has evolved. Table 3.1 gives definitions of an oncogene at several points in time over the last 25 years. Shortly after the discovery of oncogenes and up to the 1970s, an oncogene was a *viral* gene that possibly caused cancer in animals. For a while, RNA retroviruses were thought to be the principal cause of cancer. In the late 1970s we were startled to learn that the virus actually "caught" the gene from animals, not the other way around. It was discovered that for every viral oncogene, there exists a homologous cellular gene "proto-oncogene" whose normal function relates to control of cell growth. Retroviruses just borrow the gene from cells as a key to unlock the cell division cycle. This can lead to a proliferation of infected cells. Viral induced proliferation however is only one mechanism for neoplastic transformation of cells.

In the 1980s confusion arose because of the inclusion of other important cancer associated genes under a broader definition of oncogene. Genes such as *RB* and p53 were discovered that act as inhibitors of tumor formation in their normal state. Mutation of these genes destroys this inhibition. Mutated forms of p53 are very common in tumors and an important event in multistep carcinogenesis. For a few years, these genes were

Table 3.1. Historic definitions of an oncogene.

"Hypothetical viral genetic material carrying the potential of cancer and passed from parent to offspring" (*Dorland's Illustrated Medical Dictionary*. 25th ed. Philadelphia: W.B. Saunders; 1974:1081.)

"Many tumor viruses carry one or several genetic loci (known as oncogenes) that are directly and solely responsible for neoplastic transformation of the host cell" (Alberts B et al. *Molecular Biology of the Cell*. New York: Garland; 1983:623.)

"Normal cellular genes (proto-oncogenes) controlling growth, development, and differentiation that somehow become misdirected (i.e., converted to oncogenes) in the neoplastic cancer cell" (Burck KB, Liu ET, Larrick JW. *Oncogenes. An Introduction to the Concept of Cancer Genes*. New York: Springer-Verlag; 1988:1.)

"Genes capable of inducing neoplastic transformation are termed *oncogenes*." (Tronick SR, Aaronson SA. Oncogenes. In: Cossman J, ed. *Molecular Genetics in Cancer Diagnosis*. New York: Elsevier; 1990: 29.)

"A gene capable under certain conditions of causing the initial and continuing conversion of normal cells into cancer cells. The term may be used to denote such a gene occurring in a viral oncogene (v-*onc*) or a cellular gene derived from alteration of a proto-oncogene (c-*onc*)." (*Dorland's Illustrated Medical Dictionary*. 28th ed. Philadelphia: W.B. Saunders; 1994:1177.)

"Any of a family of genes which under normal circumstances code for proteins involved in cell growth or regulation but may foster malignant processes if mutated or activated by contact with retrovirus." (*Stedman's Concise Medical Dictionary*. 3rd ed. Baltimore: Williams and Wilkins; 1997.)

---

called "**antioncogenes**" because they inhibited tumor growth. The term antioncogene has subsequently been replaced with the term "tumor suppressor gene." Tumor suppressor genes however do not have a homologue in a retrovirus.

Serious controversy continues among cancer researchers as to the use of the term oncogene. A researcher in the field of retroviruses probably continues to use the term in the tightly defined sense requiring the existence of both a viral and cellular form. Many others use the term oncogene in a broader generic sense to include all genes involved in cell growth that when mutated are associated with the formation of tumors.

As a note of caution, before we continue let's take another look at Table 3.1. We need to reflect on how much our definition of an oncogene has changed. Certainly the definition continues to be refined. We can enjoy the excitement of our growing detailed knowledge of the molecular biology of cancer, but we must remember it is far from complete.

Proto-Oncogene Functions

A **proto-oncogene** is the normal form of an oncogene. This is the form the gene takes as it carries out its usual physiologic functions in a cell. When the gene is mutated, so as to cause uncontrolled cell proliferation, we drop the "proto-" and call it an oncogene. The physiologic function of proto-oncogenes is the **cell signaling pathway**. This is the pathway by which a cell receives the stimulus to undergo mitosis or apoptosis. Figure 3.1 is a schematic diagram of some of the steps in the cell signal pathway, beginning at the external surface of the cell. A growth factor present in the blood or on the surface of another cell binds to its specific receptor. This binding changes the shape of the receptor, affecting its intracytoplasmic piece. This shape change carries the signal generated by the growth factor across the cell membrane without the growth factor actually entering the cell. The signal is further propagated through the cytoplasm to the nucleus by one or more intermediate molecules such as the G proteins. The signal finally reaches the nucleus, binding to DNA at a specific transcription site. The DNA signal causes the cell to alter its proliferative state; by dividing, becoming quiescent, or destroying itself via apoptosis.

Each of the proteins that are part of this cell signal pathway is the product of proto-oncogenes. If a mutation occurs that makes the protein "hyper-"functional, then the proto-oncogene is converted to an oncogene. Table 3.2 provides an overview, listing classes of oncogenes corresponding to the steps in the cell signaling pathway shown in Figure 3.1.

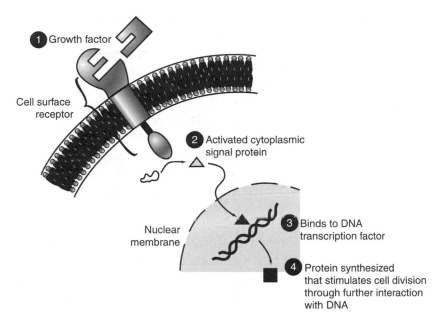

FIGURE 3.1. The cell signaling pathway receives external signals that are carried stepwise into the nucleus. The endpoint of the signal is an interaction with DNA affecting cell growth.

A few examples of each class are given in this table. Let us look at each class in more detail.

Growth Factors and Cell Surface Receptors

A cell communicates with the outside world predominantly through the receptors on its surface. Signals are received; the cell modifies its function, and sometimes sends out its own signal. We are interested in those signals that cause a cell to change its proliferation. There are very many

Table 3.2. Classes of oncogenes.

Location	Examples
External to the cell growth factors	Platelet derived growth factor (*PDGF*)
	Colony stimulating factors (M-*CSF*)
Cell membrane growth factor receptors	Epidermal growth factor receptor (*ERB*-B)
	Colony stimulating factor-1 receptor (*FMS*)
Cell cytoplasm G proteins	*GSP*
Cell nucleus transcription factors	*myc*

growth factors and a corresponding number of growth factor receptors. Without this diversity, the communication between cells would be very limited. Figure 3.2 is a more detailed schematic drawing of a growth factor receptor. The receptor consists of at least one, but usually several, proteins. Each protein is the product of a different proto-oncogene. Cell surface receptors have an external portion outside the membrane that is configured to a very specific function. The receptor binds just a certain type of growth factor, and only under specific physiologic conditions. The growth factor receptor might be designed so that it is sensitive to soluble proteins dissolved in the blood and extracellular fluid. Another receptor may only react to growth factors present on the surface of cells, requiring cell-to-cell contact to establish a signal.

Figure 3.2 demonstrates a receptor that goes all the way through the cytoplasmic membrane. Some growth factor receptors are more complicated than that. A receptor can be composed of a group of molecules that take the signal through the cell membrane in stages. However, all receptors or receptor complexes must have an external, transmembrane, and intracytoplasmic domain. The external domain establishes a stereo-chemical site that binds only to specific growth factors. A small change in either the receptor or the growth factor, and the two may no longer be a fit. The transmembrane portion of the receptor, like all molecules that pierce the cell membrane, must not allow undesired leakage of ions into or out of the cell. The intracytoplasmic portion of the receptor is a molecule that changes its functional activity when a growth factor binds to the exterior. Frequently this molecule is a tyrosine kinase (see later Table 3.3). The kinase molecule passes the signal on by converting a substrate molecule within the cytoplasm.

These receptors are beautiful molecular machines. I imagine a cell with all kinds of antennae sticking out; each tuned to its own growth factor. A

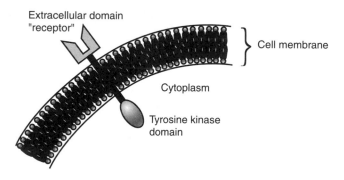

FIGURE 3.2. A cell surface receptor is composed of both extracellular, transmembrane, and intracytoplasmic protein.

Table 3.3. A somewhat comprehensive list of oncogenes.

Growth factors	Apoptosis/Cell cycle
INT-2	*BAX*
SIS	*CYCLIN* D1
Growth factor receptor	*bcl2*
erb B	Fusion genes
FMS	*ALL/MLL*
her-2/neu	*BCR*
KIT	*PBX*1
MAS	*RAR*a
MET	Others
ROS	*AKT*
RET	*CBL*
SEA	*CRK*
TRK	*EYK*
Signal transducers	*FIM* 1,2
ABL	*FPS*
FES	*HST*
FGR	*INT*-1,2
GSP	*MAF*
GLP	*MIL*
LCK	*QIN*
MOS	
PIM	
RAF	
H-*ras*	
K-*ras*	
N-*ras*	
src	
YES	
DNA binding	
erb A	
ETS	
fos	
jun	
myb	
C-*myc*	
L-*myc*	
N-*myc*	
REL	
SKI	

cell can easily have thousands of receptors! These growth factor receptors are not static. They may be removed by external factors that cleave them off. The cell may down regulate a specific receptor to a nonfunctional state. The cell retains the option of turning the receptor back on later. One growth factor may be a signal for the cell to synthesize another class of receptor. For example, breast epithelial cells change their growth factor receptors in response to cycling estrogen levels.

The cell signal pathway in cancer cells fails due to a mutation in one or more of the proto-oncogenes that code for the component proteins of the pathway. Usually the mutation produces a hyper-functioning protein. As an example, consider a mutation in the proto-oncogene that codes for the intracytoplasmic tyrosine kinase piece of the receptor. The mutation makes the kinase function so efficiently that it sends its signal on to the cytoplasm all the time, even without a growth factor binding to the exterior. A cell with this mutation would receive a signal to proliferate independent of its growth factor.

One of many examples of a hyper-functioning tyrosine kinase in a cancer cell is the mutation associated with chronic myeloid leukemia (CML, see also Chapter 7). In CML cells, some as yet unknown event causes chromosomal breaks. Chromosomes 9 and 22 switch pieces of their long ends resulting in a translocation, the **t(9;22) Philadelphia chromosome**. The translocation results in an oncogene called abelson (*ABL*) being fused with a gene called *BCR*. The proto-oncogene product of *ABL* is a tyrosine kinase molecule of molecular weight 190 kd. The fusion with *BCR* results in an oncogene, *BCR/ABL*, whose protein is a 210-kd tyrosine kinase. The *BCR/ABL* fusion protein is hyper-efficient and results in an unregulated turn on of the cell signal pathway.

Cytoplasmic and Nuclear Components of Cell Signaling Pathway

Following the cell signal pathway in Figure 3.1 further, we reach proteins that carry the signal through the cytoplasm and into the nucleus. The **G proteins** are a class of onco-proteins that convert from an inactive to active form upon receiving the correct signal from the intracytoplasmic domain of a growth factor receptor. One of the proto-oncogenes coding a G protein is *GSP*. *GSP* is subject to point mutations. These are single nucleotide switches in a gene sequence that cause hyper-efficiency of the mutated protein. Thyroid tumors are an example of a cancer associated with *GSP* point mutations.

The G proteins and all other signals must eventually effect a change in gene expression by binding to DNA. The *myc* proto-oncogene is a good example of a DNA binding protein at the end of the pathway. The level of *myc* protein affects whether a cell will be stimulated to mitosis. The final control of proliferation by a direct binding protein such as *myc* is more complicated than an on-off switch. The amount of *myc* protein is counter-balanced by other proteins such as p53 that retard cell division (as we will discuss again in Chapter 4). However, when *myc* is mutated to a high level of expression, a cell is under a strong stimulus to divide. An example of a mutation of the *myc* proto-oncogene is the pediatric cancer, neuroblastoma. In neuroblastoma, N-*myc* (one of a family of *myc* genes) is amplified within the genome. Amplified means that there are multiple copies of the gene. When multiple gene copies are present, the gene is hyper-efficient leading to too much N-*myc* protein and a stimulus to unregulated division. The number of copies of the N-*myc* gene in biopsy samples of neuroblastoma (which can be measured in the laboratory) helps determine the biological aggressiveness of that patient's tumor.

Apoptosis, Cell Cycle, and Other Oncogenes

Not all oncogenes are associated with the cell signaling pathway. A very important group are those genes that influence the cell cycle via the cyclin proteins and through apoptosis. The Cyclin D1 (formerly called *bcl-1* or *PRAD*) gene is an important example. In Chapter 7, we will look at mantle cell lymphoma. This is a cancer that results from a translocation that places the Cyclin D1 gene within the immunoglobulin gene. The result is a hyper-expression of Cyclin D1 protein and a forcing of malignant lymphocytes into the cell cycle. Later in Chapter 7, we will examine follicular lymphoma and *bcl-2*. Follicular lymphoma results from a translocation of *bcl-2* also into the immunoglobulin gene. The result is a deregulation of *bcl-2* expression with suppression of normal apoptosis.

Table 3.3 is a somewhat comprehensive list of oncogenes, including all of the examples and classes that we have discussed, as well as "others." A comprehensive table of oncogenes will always be under revision. Some oncogenes will later be reclassified as tumor suppressor genes. Others will be dropped with new ones added, as we better understand the genes that control cell growth and maturation.

Oncogenes and Clonal Proliferation

Before we go any further, I want to connect our growing theory of the action of oncogenes with the development of tumors. We have considered a few examples of how loss of the normal proto-oncogene function in the cell signaling pathway results in a stimulus to proliferate (e.g., *BCR/ABL* in CML and N-*myc* in neuroblastoma). I think we are ready to look at this whole problem more generally. Figure 3.3 demonstrates several models in which a mutated proto-oncogene results in a **clonal** proliferation of cells. A clone is a group of genetically identical cells. We

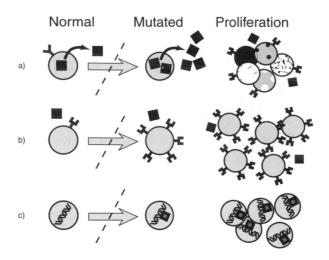

FIGURE 3.3. Mutated oncogenes can lead to clonal proliferation by several mechanisms: (a) mutated cell loses its receptor that provides negative feedback control for growth factor production. The cell overproduces growth factor causing polyclonal proliferation in adjacent nonmutated growth factor sensitive cells. This is a benign self- limiting neoplasm; (b) mutated cell produces too many growth factor receptors and is ultrasensitive to growth stimulation. This cell and its progeny proliferate as a clonal tumor, but the tumor is still sensitive to the external growth factor; and (c) mutated cell produces too much growth factor to which the cell itself is sensitive. The cell and its progeny proliferate as a clonal tumor independent of external factors.

begin life as a single cell, the fertilized zygote. Every cell in our body is essentially a clone of this original cell. Some genetic remodeling does occur during our lives that produces subclones. For example, a lymphocyte exposed to a specific antigen rearranges its immunoglobulin genes to produce a corresponding specific antibody. That lymphocyte divides and produces a subclone of lymphocytes, all producing the specific antibody. A mutation in a proto-oncogene results in a cell with a proliferation advantage. That cell reproduces itself into a neoplastic clone, and this is the start of cancer. The neoplastic clone is very susceptible to further mutation, generating subclones. The most rapidly dividing (or surviving) subclone will always come to the fore.

Let us look at several models of the production of neoplastic clones as schematized in Figure 3.3. In the first model, a mutated cell loses its "Y" shaped *inhibitory* receptor for growth factor production. The cell has permanently lost any inhibition and oversecretes growth factor. Nearby, nonmutated cells sensitive to the growth factor proliferate. Their proliferation is limited by a relatively small excess supply of growth factor. This is a model of a benign self-limiting, nonclonal proliferation of cells.

The second model in Figure 3.3 demonstrates a true clonal neoplasm. Here, the mutated cell produces too many growth factor receptors. This cell and all its progeny are hypersensitive to growth stimulation. The mutated cell proliferates as a clonal tumor, but the tumor is still sensitive to the external growth factor. Removing the growth factor stops growth of the tumor. Thus, removal of the growth factor, if possible, would be a useful form of therapy for this type of tumor.

In the third model, all limits on the growth of the neoplasm are removed. This time, the mutation results in a cell that produces too much of its *own* growth factor. The cell and its progeny proliferate as a clonal tumor independent of external factors.

These three models demonstrate how different mutations in the cell signal pathway produce neoplasms with very different growth properties. The first model is not actually a neoplasm, because the proliferating cells are not clonal. The third model is a highly malignant tumor. We will return to the molecular events that dictate the behavior of tumors in Chapter 5, when we consider the multiple events necessary to convert a normal cell into a cancer.

Mutations that Convert Proto-Oncogenes to Oncogenes

We now have an idea of the cell signal pathway, the proto-oncogenes that control its function, and how mutation to an oncogene results in a clonal tumor. But how do these oncogene mutations come about? There are a number of mechanisms creating mutations that activate an oncogene such as: point mutation, insertion/deletion mutation, chromosomal translocation, and gene amplification. We will consider mutations in more detail in Chapter 5 when we discuss carcinogenesis. However, a few examples of mutations in this chapter will help us understand oncogenes.

Point Mutation

A very direct example of oncogene activation is point mutation. The switch of a single base changes the codon for one amino acid in the protein. If this switch makes the protein nonfunctional, that's the end of the story. No proliferative advantage results from inactivation of an oncogene. If the point mutation results in a hyper-functioning protein, then we have proliferation. An example is the *ras* family of oncogenes (N-*ras*, H-*ras*, K-*ras*). Within *ras* genes, a point mutation at codon 12, 59, or 61 results in a hyper-function of the protein. The *ras* proteins are part of the intracytoplasmic portion of the cell signal pathway. *ras* mutations are frequent in lung, colon, and pancreas cancers. A point mutation in *ras* is one important step in the multistep formation of a cancer. We will look at the genetic map of K-*ras* at the end of this chapter; and *ras* will reappear in Chapter 5 (multistep carcinogenesis) and Chapter 8 (colon cancer).

Retroviruses

The biology of **retroviruses** is an important topic for us. The insertion of the genome of a retrovirus into human DNA during the life cycle of the virus is a potential mutagenic event. Early experiments in which it was noted that infection with a retrovirus transformed mammalian cells in culture led to the discovery of oncogenes. Ironically, we now know that few human cancers are directly related to retrovirus infection. Retroviruses have a genome consisting of two copies of a single RNA strand* (diploid genome). The genome is typically 3500 to 9000 bp. Three important genes, *GAG, POL,* and *ENV* occur in all retroviruses. *GAG* codes for the protein coat or capsid of the virus. *POL* codes for a **reverse transcriptase** enzyme that allows for the viral RNA to be converted to DNA when it is within the cell. *ENV* codes for proteins in the envelope that surrounds the capsid.

Figure 3.4 is a map of the genome of a specific retrovirus, the Rous sarcoma virus (RSV). The RNA genome begins with a cap at the 5′ end. The three viral genes follow. A fourth gene *src* is a **viral oncogene** that produces a protein capable of transforming cells, forcing them into pro-

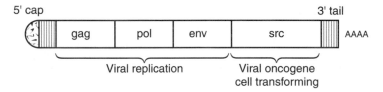

FIGURE 3.4. A genetic map of the Rous sarcoma virus, RSV, contains the three genes common to all retroviruses (*GAG,POL,ENV*) and a viral oncogene, *src*, with cell transforming ability.

---

*At the beginning of Chapter 1, we defined a gene as being a piece of DNA. Here is an exception. Retroviruses use RNA as their genetic material. However, as we shall see, when a retrovirus infects a cell, it causes its genome to be reverse transcribed to a DNA copy.

liferation. Within the virus, this gene is called v- *src*. The corresponding proto-oncogene, c-*src* was first discovered in chickens that developed sarcomas when infected with the retrovirus. Not all retroviruses carry a viral oncogene. For example, the human immunodeficiency virus, HIV, has only the *GAG, POL* and *ENV* genes.

The genome of a retrovirus is very minimal. The virus has a life cycle within the cell that takes advantage of the cell's genes to do what the virus cannot do alone. Figure 3.5 demonstrates the life cycle of a retrovirus. The virus has a glycoprotein envelope (*env*) surrounding a capsid (*gag*) that in turn encloses the RNA genome. In order to infect a cell, the virus must attach to the surface. The virus binds to cell surface receptors by having its envelope proteins imitate a match to a normal cell receptor. The virus can only infect the cells that express this receptor. HIV binds to a complex of the CD4 and CXCR-4 receptors on the surface of T-

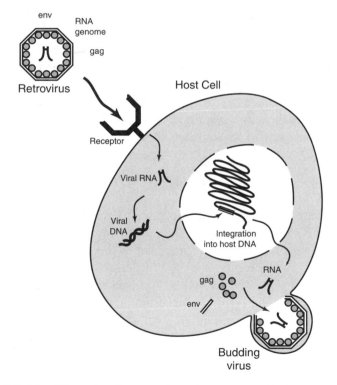

FIGURE 3.5. The life cycle of a retrovirus shows the multiple steps where: the virus binds to a cell surface receptor; viral RNA enters the cytoplasm; is copied into DNA; integrates into the host DNA; and eventually propagates budding off new virus particles.

helper lymphocytes. The RSV retrovirus binds to specific receptors on chicken cells. After the virus enters the cell, its RNA genome is released. The viral *POL* gene serves as a template for the cell cytoplasm to make the reverse transcriptase enzyme that copies the viral RNA into double-stranded DNA. The *POL* enzyme is called reverse transcriptase because it works in the opposite direction of normal transcription, making a DNA copy of RNA. Reverse transcriptase is the enzyme unique to all retroviruses. They must have it, because their genome is written in RNA. Many of the antiviral drugs for HIV are directed against this unique enzyme.

The viral derived DNA integrates into DNA of the host nucleus. It is just a smidgen of material in the huge human genome. But like one extra period in a paragraph, it can alter the meaning. If the viral DNA contains a transforming oncogene, the cell may be driven into proliferation by the insertion of the retrovirus. This occurs in the case of RSV infecting chicken cells. The virus reproduces itself using the cell's machinery. New viral particles are assembled inside the cell and then bud off the cell surface, as is shown in Figure 3.5.

It is the insertion of the viral genome into the cell's DNA that interests us the most. It is at this moment that a retrovirus has the potential to mutate a proto-oncogene. The viral genome now transcribed into DNA inserts into the cell's nuclear DNA by a process of cutting, insertion, and splicing. These events carry the potential to alter the genome of the cell. The insertion of the virus is a mutagenic event that can convert the cellular proto-oncogene to its activated form.

Genetic Structure of Oncogenes

Before we leave this chapter on oncogenes, I would like to look at a genetic map of K-*ras* in more detail. Oncogenes are relatively short and simple genes. Figure 3.6 shows the gene map of the viral and cellular forms of K-*ras*. The viral gene is only 900 bp long. The cellular proto-oncogene K-*ras* is slightly spread out, or "un-packed" into four exons spanning about 25 kb. The open reading frame codes for a 189 amino acid, 21-kd protein. At several points, the *ras* genome is susceptible to point mutations that render the protein hyper-functional. Codons 12, 59, and 61 are shown in Figure 3.6 with their normal nonmutated base sequences. These are the "hot-spots" in *ras*.

The genetic structure of the other members of the *ras* family, H-*ras* and N- *ras* is quite similar to that shown in Figure 3.6. All oncogenes are relatively simple. This is probably because they must be compact enough to fit into a viral form of the gene. Another property of oncogenes that is

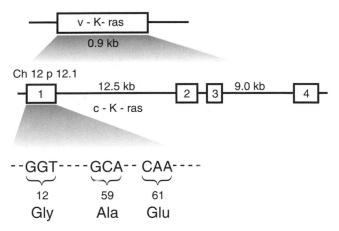

FIGURE 3.6. A genetic map demonstrates the similarity of viral and cellular proto-oncogene forms of K-*ras*. Three exons (#12,59,61) are the sites of point mutations that activate the oncogene to a hyper-functional state.

intriguing is their similarity throughout the animal kingdom. The genetic sequence of the human c-*myc* oncogene is only 1% different than a mouse. Yet, there is a 10% difference in the base pairs of the hemoglobin genes in man and the mouse. Why is there this conservation of the oncogene structure throughout evolution? Perhaps oncogenes are already in a compact, essential form so that most mutations do not survive. Another possible mechanism is a "correction" occurs when the gene passes through a viral form. There is still much to be discovered about oncogenes.

Summary

Oncogenes are normal human growth control genes that have mutated to become hyper-functional. In their normal form, proto-oncogenes code for the components of the cell signaling pathway. This pathway is the means by which a cell receives outside signals that direct its proliferation and differentiation. Cancer cells have mutation in this pathway that causes them to misread or become entirely independent of these outside signals.

References

Burck KB, Liu ET, Larrick JW. *Oncogenes. An Introduction to the Concept of Cancer Genes*. New York: Springer-Verlag, 1988.

Cancer Genome Anatomy Project (CGAP). http://www.ncbi.nlm.nih.gov/ncic-gap. Also http://www.ncbi.nlm.nih.gov/science96/gene?HRAS

Tronick SR, Aaronson SA. Oncogenes. In: Cossman J, ed. *Molecular Genetics in Cancer Diagnosis*. New York: Elsevier; 1990:29–48.

Weinberg RA. Molecular Mechanisms of Carcinogenesis. In: Leder P, Clayton DA, Rubenstein E, eds. *Introduction to Molecular Medicine*. New York: Scientific American; 1994:253–276.

Tumor Suppressor Genes

Overview

"Oncogenes promote cell growth; tumor suppressor genes inhibit it."

This is an oversimplification of the myriad of molecular functions under the control of these genes. Proto-oncogenes, as we discussed in the last chapter, encode for proteins in the cell signaling pathway and apoptosis. When mutated into oncogenes, their function results in an unregulated stimulation of cell division. Mutated oncogenes act in a dominant genetic mode, producing an abnormal phenotype, even though a second allele of the gene is not mutated. Tumor suppressor genes (at one time called antioncogenes*) have the normal physiologic role of retarding cell division. Tumor suppressor genes differ from oncogenes in several other ways besides their opposing effects on cell division. Tumor suppressor genes do not exist in a viral form, as is the case for oncogenes. This should not be surprising. A retrovirus benefits from carrying an oncogene along in its genome to promote division in cells it infects. There would be no benefit to a virus in carrying a copy of a tumor suppressor gene to retard cell division. Tumor suppressor genes work with the DNA repair system, so necessary in maintaining the stability of the genome. Tumor suppressor genes in mutated form can be passed on as germline heritable DNA defects. They are the cause of the syndromes of genetic predisposition to cancer. However, tumor suppressor gene mutations occur more commonly as sporadic somatic cell mutations in nonfamilial cancers. Tumor suppressor genes are recessive. Both copies of the gene must be mutated to produce the phenotype: failure to inhibit growth of damaged cells. Table 4.1 lists these contrasting features of oncogenes and tumor suppressor genes.*

Tumor suppressor genes, although recessive, become inactivated more commonly than would be expected due to an important genetic mechanism, loss of heterozygosity (LOH). We look at LOH in some detail. This knowledge is part of our understanding of cancer as a multi-

step process. We then look at some examples of tumor suppressor genes including RB1 and p53 in some detail. The p53 tumor suppressor gene plays a pivotal role as a final common step in carcinogenesis. Mutations in p53 are found in over 50% of human cancers. This chapter concludes with a repeated cautionary statement: there is a lot we do not yet know about this subject.

Table 4.1. Characteristics of oncogenes and tumor suppressor genes.

Oncogene	Tumor suppressor gene
Exists in a viral form	No viral counterpart
Acts as a dominant trait, single allele mutation in tumors	Acts as a recessive trait, two alleles mutated in tumors
Gene protein functions directly in regulation of cell growth, promotes	Gene protein functions directly in regulation of cell growth, inhibits
Mutated to hyper-function in tumors	Mutated to inactivation in tumors
Not inherited as germ line mutation, acquired as a somatic mutation	Inherited as a trait or acquired as a somatic mutation

Genetics of Tumor Suppressor Genes and Loss of Heterozygosity (LOH)

Recall from Chapter 1 our first gene, *BRCA*1, the breast and ovary cancer susceptibility gene. Women born with an inherited defect in one of the two copies of *BRCA*1 have a high probability of developing breast cancer in their mid-life years. This epidemiological fact implies that just one copy of the *BRCA*1 gene is not sufficient to hold breast cancer in check. Mutations in breast epithelium pile up over the years. The function of *BRCA*1 is to hold mutated cells from proliferating into tumors. Sometime in 40 or so years, a woman born with only one normal *BRCA*1 gene must experience a loss of that remaining normal gene. This phenomenon is called loss of heterozygosity.

Loss of heterozygosity, or **LOH** in genetic jargon, is an extremely important genetic mechanism leading to the inactivation of tumor suppressor genes. A person who has inherited damage to one of the two alleles for a tumor suppressor gene might expect to live their life tumor free, under protection of the other allele. After all, the chances of a random mutation knocking out the other allele are infinitesimal, one in a million or less. Yet we know that loss of the second allele does occur. Loss of heterozygosity is the mechanism whereby the second allele is damaged with high frequency.

Figure 4.1 demonstrates how LOH leads to the common occurrence of tumor in a person with an inherited cancer predisposition. For this example, we will consider *RB*1; the retinoblastoma associated tumor suppressor gene. At the top of the figure is the genotype of a male who has inherited one mutated *RB*1 tumor suppressor gene on chromosome 13. By the convention of genetic pedigrees, we indicate a male with a square and the partial shading means that the subject is a heterozygote. The defective copy of the gene is marked as − and the normal or "wild-type" allele as +. The two copies of the chromosome 13 are designated *a* and *b* in order that we may distinguish them in subsequent genetic mixes. The proband* in this example has the genotype *RB*1 +/− in every cell in his body except within haploid sperm cells which are either *RB*1 + or −.

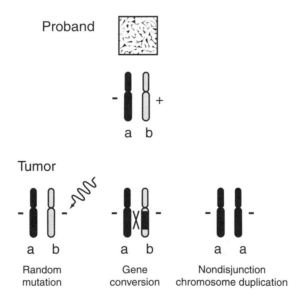

FIGURE 4.1. In a proband with a hereditary mutation in *RB*1, several paths lead to loss of heterozygosity of the second allele resulting in familial retinoblastoma.

Proband is the term for a person under genetic study. If that person is ill, it is more appropriate to call him or her a *patient*.

In the lower half of Figure 4.1, I show three different possible tumor genotypes for a retinoblastoma developing in our proband. Remember that these are *tumor* genotypes. The additional mutations occur only in tumor cells. The genotype of the individual in every remaining cell except for the tumor remains unchanged.

In the left hand panel of Figure 4.1, the second allele on chromosome 13^b has been damaged by a random mutation. This is the least likely way to acquire LOH in this situation. This is the "one-in-a-million" random mutation.

The center panel of Figure 4.1 shows a second tumor genotype with a and b copies of chromosome 13, but now both alleles are mutated. The wild-type allele on chromosome b has undergone gene conversion. Damage somewhere near the *RB*1 allele on chromosome b occurred. The cell attempts to repair itself. The damaged DNA on b is compared by base pairing with the undamaged but mutated copy on chromosome a. The cell's DNA repair mechanism tries to repair the damage, unfortunately using the mutant copy as reference. The normal allele on b is converted to the mutant allele.

The right hand panel of Figure 4.1 demonstrates a third way in which LOH can occur. The tumor cell is shown with two mutated *RB*1 alleles, but both are on chromosome 13^a. Chromosome 13^b has been entirely lost. The loss of 13^b occurred at mitosis secondary to nondisjunction of the two chromosomes 13 with unequal sharing. One daughter cell got two copies, and the other got zero copies of 13^b. The cell that got zero copies of 13^b reduplicated its copy of 13^a to compensate for loss of a chromosome. This leads to the genotype shown of *RB*1 $-/-$.

There are additional mechanisms for LOH beyond these three examples. But, all paths lead to the same result. The genotype *RB*1 $+/-$ is converted to *RB*1 $-/-$ (or *RB*1 $-/$) with higher frequency than expected based on random mutation. When we do genotyping of retinoblastomas, we find that the two mutated copies of chromosome 13 are almost always the exact same mutation. It is very unusual to find two different random mutations as shown in the left hand panel of Figure 4.1. Loss of tumor suppressor gene function is about 1000 times more common due to LOH than would be expected on the basis of a second random mutation. Without LOH, complete failure of tumor suppressor gene function would be very rare. The irony is that LOH is a result of the cell's attempt to repair DNA damage. Most of the time this repair works. If a portion of a chromosome is damaged, copying the undamaged portion on the other chromosome makes sense. It backfires when the cell copies a recessive mutation in a tumor suppressor gene.

To stress that point, let's leave cancer genetics for a moment and consider a comparable problem in "classical" genetics. A person born with sickle cell trait has two alleles, A and S, in every cell. In the bone marrow as red cells are produced, both hemoglobin A and S are synthesized. A red cell with a 50:50 mix of A and S functions normally. If LOH occurred in a bone marrow cell leading to that one cell losing its copy of A, all the red cells produced by that precursor would have only hemoglobin S. These red cells would function poorly, but the situation would be undetectable from a clinical point of view. The bone marrow cell with LOH produces only a fraction of the blood cells in the body. The level of hemoglobin S in the proband would not measurably increase. The difference in cancer is that we are dealing with mutations that lead to an increase in the number of damaged cells. The mutated cells have a selective advantage. Therefore, the damaged cells outgrow the normal cells, and this leads to a tumor. Cancer is the result of damage to DNA that leads to loss of control of cell proliferation.

The majority of cancers demonstrate mutations in a tumor suppressor gene. However, most cancers are not derived from a hereditary predisposition to cancer. Figure 4.2 demonstrates the much more common genotype of a cancer occurring solely as the result of a somatic mutation. The proband at the top of the figure is a woman with two normal copies of *RB*1. In the convention of genetic pedigrees this woman is shown as an unshaded (unaffected) circle. A random mutation, depicted in the middle of the figure, creates a cell with a mutated *RB*1 allele. The genotype of every other cell in the woman remains unchanged. Only a single cell has mutated. However, this cell is now a possible source of a future tumor if through LOH it loses the remaining normal allele. This cell is a premalignant clone. Figure 4.2 is similar to Figure 4.1, except for the intermediate step of a random mutation creating a premalignant clone. This additional step in the process is what makes tumors less common in people without an inherited mutation in a tumor suppressor gene. Families with a hereditary mutation in *RB*1 have frequent occurrence of retinoblastoma. Without an inherited *RB*1 mutation, retinoblastoma is rare. Women with an inherited *BRCA*1 mutation have a 60% to 85% risk of breast cancer. Women without a *BRCA*1 mutation have an 11% risk.

Function of Tumor Suppressor Genes

We currently understand the function of tumor suppressor genes only partially. I cannot construct for you an organized set of functions like the cell signaling pathway that explained proto-oncogenes. Table 4.2 lists ex-

Table 4.3. Characteristics of hereditary versus sporadic retinoblastoma.

	Hereditary	Sporadic
Clinical		
Ocular tumors	Multiple, bilateral	Single
Onset	Very early	Later
Additional cancers	High risk, sarcomas	No increased risk
Genetic		
% of tumors	40	60
RB genotype	+/−	+/+
Family history	Usual	Negative
	50% of offspring affected	

tosomal recessive, but the phenotype behaves as autosomal dominant due to LOH. The frequency of the *RB* +/− genotype in the general population is very low. Yet, these individuals account for nearly half of the cases of retinoblastoma. This is very different from the genetics of *BRCA*1 and breast cancer where the incidence of the +/− genotype is 1%, yet those individuals with an inherited mutation account for only 5% of breast cancers. The reasons for vastly different behavior of the genetics of different tumor suppressor genes is partially explained by the fact that they are only one step in multistep carcinogenesis (as we shall see in more detail in the next chapter).

The *RB*1 protein, designated pRB-105, has a central role in the control of the cell division cycle. *RB*1 and p53 proteins are the major brakes on progression through the cell cycle. The *RB*1 protein is progressively phosphorylated beginning in S phase, and then dephosphorylated in M and G1. The protein in its dephosphorylated form acts through transcription factors to block the activation of genes necessary to S phase. For example, the transcription of c-*myc* and c-*myb* oncoproteins can be inhibited by *RB*1. Although the cell cycle progresses in a regular clock-like fashion, *RB*1 can slow the clock down particularly around the start of S phase.

Figure 4.3 is another representation of the cell division cycle, like that shown in Figure 2.1. I have now added the points at which the tumor suppressor genes *RB* and p53 interact with cell proliferation. *RB* acts as a brake slowing the cycle near the start of S phase. p53 acts as a brake or a switch at the G1 checkpoint. If DNA damage is detected, p53 holds the cell up until repairs are completed. If damage cannot be repaired, p53 can lead to apoptosis, causing the cell to suicide. The *bcl*-2 onco-

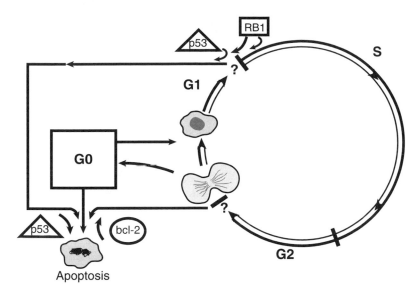

FIGURE 4.3. The *RB* and p53 tumor suppressor genes interact with the cell division cycle at several points.

gene produces a protein that overrides some of the signals leading to apoptosis. In Figure 4.3, *bcl-2* is shown as an antagonist to p53.

p53

The importance of the p53 tumor suppressor gene has attracted great attention. *Newsweek* magazine named it the "Molecule of the Year" in 1996. Mutations in the p53 gene are found in 50% of human cancers. The common involvement of p53 in cancer has led to research focused on restoring p53 function in tumor cells. When radiation or chemotherapy damages a tumor cell, the normal p53 gene induces apoptosis as one of the mechanisms for killing the cell. Without p53 function, apoptosis is less likely to occur. A p53 deficient cell damaged by therapy persists with its additional burden of DNA damage. This cell becomes a possible source of further tumor mutations. We will discuss experimental treatment based on restoring the p53 gene in several of the chapters in Part II of this book. Clinical trials are directed at: (a) direct gene transfer of nonmutated p53 DNA into tumor cells; (b) antibodies against mutated p53 protein; and (c) vaccines that kill cells without p53 function.

Figure 4.4 is a schematic diagram of the p53 gene that is located on the short arm of chromosome 17 (17p13.1) and spans 20 kb. The gene is made up of 11 exons that produce an mRNA transcript of 2800 bp. The mRNA

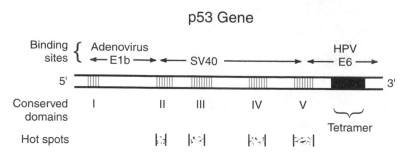

FIGURE 4.4. A gene map of p53 shows several hot spots for mutation. Viral proteins that bind to functional areas within the gene inhibit p53.

translates into a 393 amino acid protein of 53 kd. There are five domains (indicated as I through V) within the gene that are highly conserved, being nearly the same sequence in the p53 gene equivalent of many different animals. The central portion of the gene, closely correlated with the conserved domains, contains mutational hot spots. Of the thousands of mutations that have been mapped in p53 genes isolated from human tumors, a high frequency occurs within these hot spots. The function of the p53 protein is easily disrupted at these points.

Near the 3′ end of the gene is a region responsible for a portion of the protein that participates in the tetramerization of the p53 molecule. Normal p53 protein is a complex of four chains. If one of the two p53 alleles is mutated, mutant chains may mix with wild-ype chains and form a partially defective protein. By this mechanism, some mutations of p53 act as dominant, rather than the typically recessive character of tumor suppressor genes. There are several binding sites on the gene where both proteins and DNA attach, affecting the transcription of p53. Viral protein E1b from the mouse adenovirus, a protein from the SV40 virus, and E6 protein from human papilloma virus all bind to the p53 gene. As we will discuss shortly in this chapter and again in Chapter 5, the interaction of these viral proteins with tumor suppressor genes is a step in viral carcinogenesis.

The p53 protein has several functions, as we discussed in relation to Figure 4.3. p53 holds progression through the cell division cycle at the G1/S checkpoint when DNA damage is detected. This allows time for DNA repair mechanisms to correct damage before the DNA is copied in S phase. p53 can also induce apoptosis, killing a cell with extensive DNA damage. The functions of p53 are carried out through the intermediary of other genes such as p21, p16, and *WAF*1. The entire system is somewhat complex or, in a more positive sense, "rich in detail." The p53 protein is

Table 4.4. Interaction of tumor suppressor gene proteins and DNA tumor virus proteins.

Tumor suppressor gene	DNA tumor virus	Viral protein
RB1	Adenovirus, murine type 5	E1a
RB1	Papillomavirus, human especially HPV16, 18	E7
p53	Papillomavirus, human	E6
p53	Adenovirus, murine type 5	E1b
p53	Polyoma virus, simian SV40	large T

normally quite labile in the cell nucleus. When nuclear DNA is damaged, p53 protein becomes stabilized and reaches higher concentrations within the nucleus. This protein binds as a transcription factor repressing the function of other genes. The function of p53 is modulated by oncogenes such as c-*myc* and *bcl*-2. High levels of c-*myc* can override a p53 arrest of the cell cycle and *bcl*-2 can stop p53 induced apoptosis.

DNA Tumor Viruses Inactivate Tumor Suppressor Genes

Many oncogenes are present in a viral form (v-*onc*) as part of the makeup of RNA retroviruses. Tumor suppressor genes are not found in the genome of viruses. However, the protein products of several DNA tumor viruses interact with tumor suppressor genes. This leads to the virus blocking tumor suppressor gene function, i.e., viral carcinogenesis. Table 4.4 lists the interaction of mouse adenovirus, simian (monkey) tumor virus SV40, and human papilloma virus HPV with the *RB*1 and p53 proteins. We will look at the consequences of this interaction in more detail in the next chapter, and for the case of HPV in Chapter 9 on squamous cell carcinoma of the cervix. DNA tumor viruses benefit from promoting host cell proliferation. Unlike RNA retroviruses they do not carry an oncogene key to force cells to proliferate. Instead DNA tumor viruses impede the *RB*1 and p53 brakes on the cell division cycle shown in Figure 4.3.

Summary

*The web of influences on cell division becomes more and more complex.
Oncogenes promote growth. Tumor suppressor genes inhibit growth.
Oncogene and tumor suppressor genes antagonize each other in complex*

interactions. Tumor suppressor genes are recessive, but they function as "dominant" because of loss of heterozygosity when one allele is mutated. DNA tumor viruses can reversibly block tumor suppressor function.

The regulation of cell proliferation is dependent on so many factors. Cancer is a disruption of these controls at the level of the gene. Because the web of controls is so complex, there are many ways to disrupt it. In the next chapter, we will combine all of the knowledge we have acquired to this point in a multistep theory of cancer. There are so many ways in which a cell can go bad.

References

Begley S. The cancer killer. *Newsweek*, Dec 23, 1996: 42–47.

Fearon ER. Human cancer syndromes: clues to the origin and nature of cancer. *Science*. 1997;278:1043–1050.

Fearon ER, Vogelstein B. Tumor suppressor and DNA repair gene defects in human cancer. In: Holland JF, Bast RC, Morton DL, Frei E, Kufe DW, Weichselbaum RR, eds. *Cancer Medicine*. 4th ed. Baltimore: Williams and Wilkins; 1997:97–117.

Tumor Protein p53; TP53. http://www.ncbi.nlm.nih.gov/cgi-bin/SCIENCE96/gene?TP53.

Multiple Steps in the
Molecular Causes of Cancer

Overview

The cell is a beautiful machine that is very well protected from DNA mutation. A human consists of about 10^{14} of these beautiful machines, each one of which is a copy of the single-cell, fertilized zygote formed at the moment of conception. Most of the 10^{14} cells in the body are renewed continuously, raising the number of cell divisions in a human lifetime by more orders of magnitude. For example, approximately 250 billion neutrophils and an equal number of red blood cells are replaced every day of our lives by cell division. A very rough estimate is that, on the average, the cells in our body turn over once a month. At each one of these cell divisions, the 6 billion nucleotides of the human genome are faithfully copied. Again, a very rough estimate of the total number of nucleotides copied as DNA replicates during a 100-year lifetime is as follows:

(10^{14} cells/human)(10 cell divisions for each cell/year) (100 years/lifetime)(6×10^9 nucleotides/cell division)
= approximately 10^{27} nucleotides copied/human lifetime

The number 10^{27} is something only astronomers can be comfortable with. If we consider that the DNA content of a single human cell is 7×10^{-12} grams, then this calculation implies that our cells make 700 kilograms of DNA during our lifetime, copied from the original molecular speck of DNA present in the nucleus of the zygote.

Cancer occurs as the result of errors in DNA. If there were no errors in DNA, cancer would not occur. On the other hand, it is hard to imagine copying 10^{27} nucleotides over a lifetime without making many, many errors. Why don't cancerous cells arise every few minutes? The extremes—no cancer at all and cancer occurring so often as to not per-

57

mit human life—are philosophical boundaries that we can only con-template. What we do know is that cancer does occur during the life-time of about one-third of us. The incidence of cancer increases sharply with age, as demonstrated graphically in Figure 5.1 (data from Ries et al. 1996).

In this chapter, we pull together the basic science of the previous four chapters and examine cancer as a multistep process resulting from the ac-cumulation of uncorrected mutations in DNA. The activation of an onco-gene and loss of heterozygosity in a tumor suppressor gene are the first steps. We look at the causes of these mutations, the process of carcino-genesis. Chemical, radiation, and viral carcinogenesis offer specific ex-amples.

The creation of a cancer cell is not the end of the process. The malig-nant clone must establish a foothold in the body. The cancer must de-velop a blood supply through angiogenesis, overcome the immune sys-tem, and develop the ability to spread through metastasis. This chapter concludes with what I hope is a solid argument that there is no longer a clear-cut line between benign and malignant. Cancer is a multistep process

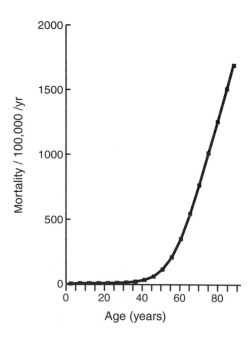

FIGURE 5.1. The death rate from cancer rises dramatically with ad-vancing age.

that presents a progressive spectrum of clinical behavior based on the stage at which it is detected.

Carcinogenesis

Carcinogenesis is a process by which agents that result in mutations lead to cancer. We have seen in Chapters 3 and 4 that this means agents that cause mutations in oncogenes and tumor suppressor genes. The list of carcinogens is very, very large. Chemicals, radiation, and viruses are the main classes of carcinogens. The potency of a particular carcinogen can be very high or quite low, and is difficult to measure in a way that is clinically relevant. Most carcinogens are measured in a single-step experimental assay. We ask, "What is the potential of a single inhaled dose of diethylnitrosamine to induce breast tumors in a rat?" How this information carries over into predicting human risk based on chronic exposure is a very difficult topic. There have been very many public scares about one chemical or another, based on poorly presented information. The brief survey of carcinogenesis that I shall present hopefully simplifies this discussion. The agents that cause mutations are many; some such as cigarette smoke are more within our ability to avoid than others.

Chemical Carcinogenesis

A chemical carcinogen damages DNA by binding to it and causing strand breaks or interfering with DNA replication, either of which can cause a mutation. Most often, the chemical carcinogen itself must be converted to an activated intermediary form in order for DNA binding to occur. Figure 5.2 lists the steps leading from exposure up through mutation. Detoxification and elimination of both the carcinogen and its intermediaries are very dose dependent. The complex between the carcinogen and DNA is called a **DNA adduct**. The DNA adduct may damage the DNA directly by single- or double-strand breakage. The adduct may also cause a chemical change in a nucleotide, such as methylation of cytosine. The damage to DNA by carcinogens may not be manifest until DNA replication occurs, at which time the adduct leads to incorrect copying near where it is bound. The nature and extent of DNA damage greatly affects the outcome. Of course, the most usual outcome is repair of the DNA damage. Or if the damage is not repaired, this is detected and the cell undergoes apoptosis. Only if the repair systems fail do we have a mutation.

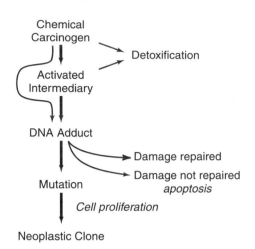

FIGURE 5.2. Chemical carcinogenesis involves multiple steps with the possibility for detoxification or repair.

The effect of chemical carcinogens is greatly modulated by other conditions. If the DNA mutation occurs in a terminally differentiated cell such as a skin keratinocyte, the result will be limited by the cell physiologically sloughing off in the near future. The same mutation occurring in an oncogene in a bone marrow stem cell will be a significant step towards developing leukemia.

Cells must undergo division in order for mutations to lead to a neoplastic clone. Effective chemical carcinogenesis frequently involves more than one compound, an **initiator** that mutates and a **promoter** that stimulates cell division. Cigarette smoke contains agents that are mutagens, as well as irritants that stimulate cell division. Testing of chemicals one at a time for carcinogenic potential does not take into account this synergistic effect. A chemical that provokes mutations in breast epithelium may be effective only when the breast is under physiologic hormonal stimulation.

Radiation Carcinogenesis

Ionizing radiation damages cells by disrupting molecular structures. The damage to molecules other than DNA is not very significant in terms of disease except at very high doses. Ionizing radiation is no different than a chemical carcinogen, except that we know rather more about the details. The nuclear age that followed the Second World War spun off a great deal of biological research on radiation effects. The military wanted to know about every aspect of this weapon, including the long term health effects. The public wanted to know of the dangers of this new form of energy.

The interaction of ionizing radiation with DNA depends on the energy of the radiation, the dose, and the type of particle (for example x-ray versus neutron beam). The most important damage to DNA is double-strand breaks. This frequently results in mutation. Based on experiments in animals and extensive data from human exposure such as the Hiroshima bomb survivors, the increased incidence of cancer following radiation can be estimated. The incidence of leukemia is doubled for every 20 cGy of radiation exposure. Other cancers have a doubling dose of about 100 cGy. Radiation can easily be detected and quantified with Geiger counters. This is not so for chemical carcinogens, most of which are invisible to us without specialized testing.

Viral Carcinogenesis

Viruses were at one time thought to be the predominant cause of cancer. Recall from Chapter 3 that oncogenes were discovered in viruses. There are many animal models of tumors in which viruses play a central role. In humans however, viral carcinogenesis has so far been found only rarely. A prime example is adult T-cell leukemia secondary to the retrovirus human T-cell leukemia virus (**HTLV-1**). HTLV-1 infection predominantly involves CD4 T-helper lymphocytes (as does infection with closely related HIV). An HTLV-1 viral protein *tax* causes an increase in the number of interleukin 2 (IL-2) receptors on infected lymphocytes. These lymphocytes are preferentially stimulated into division by the cytokine IL-2. The first step in HTLV-1 carcinogenesis is a polyclonal lymphocytosis. Later, by an unknown mechanism, a malignant clone arises from one of the stimulated lymphocytes.

Viral carcinogenesis is very different from chemical or radiation effects. Viruses damage the information within the genome by genetic mechanisms rather than a chemical disruption of the DNA. HTLV-1 produces a stimulatory signal. Other viruses may act by carrying oncogenes to an insertion point adjacent to cell proliferation genes (insertional activation).

Viruses can also cause cancer by indirect nongenetic effects. We will explore in detail in Chapter 9 the role of the human papilloma virus (HPV) in causing squamous cell carcinoma of the cervix. In Chapter 4, we discussed the interaction of the HPV E6 and E7 proteins with the *RB*1 and p53 tumor suppressor gene. This is an example of indirect viral carcinogenesis. The host cell DNA has not been irreversibly altered by mutation.

Rather, the viral protein has reversibly shut down the cell's repair system. This allows the virus to propagate in cells. If the virus had not interfered with the cell's p53 DNA repair system, the cell would consider itself damaged and would not permit DNA synthesis.

Other viruses *cause* cancer by inhibiting the immune system. Their effect is very indirect and I use the word "*cause*" with tongue in cheek. We have reached a point of sophistication in our study of cancer to know that there is no single cause. As we will discuss at the end of this chapter, the immune system is one of the last barriers that a tumor must overcome in order to spread as a lethal metastasizing cancer. Anything that chronically suppresses the immune system thus becomes a carcinogenic effect. Chronic immune suppression leads to an increased incidence of cancer as seen in HIV infected patients, patients with chronic malaria, and in patients on long term immuno-suppressive therapy.

Chemoprotection from Cancer

So called **chemoprotection** from cancer is focused on decreasing mutations due to carcinogens. A substance that converts a chemical carcinogen to an inactive form, or helps in the body's detoxification would be a chemoprotector. The formation of highly reactive chemical free radicals is a frequent first step in damage to DNA. Foods, nutritional supplements, or drugs that "absorb" free radicals fall into the class of chemoprotectors. Since carcinogenesis is dependent on so many variables, the effectiveness of chemoprotection is difficult to measure.

Other means of limiting carcinogenesis include substances such as vitamins that induce differentiation. Vitamin A will cause certain tissues to mature more rapidly. Bronchial mucosa in the lung that is irritated and has undergone metaplasia from columnar to squamous epithelium will benefit from vitamin A. In this instance, the squamous epithelium will differentiate more rapidly, sloughing off cells that might otherwise evolve from metaplastic to dysplastic. In cigarette smokers, vitamin A has the potential to work as an antipromoter of carcinogenesis. Oral contraceptives may alter the incidence of breast cancer by changing the hormonal modulation of cell proliferation in breast epithelium.

The best protection for viral associated tumors is avoidance of the virus or immunity by vaccination. Hepatitis B vaccination has lowered the incidence of hepatocellular carcinoma in China. New DNA vaccines against HPV are expected to offer protection from cervical carcinoma (see Chapters 9 and 11).

Angiogenesis

As a neoplastic clone of cells grows, it eventually reaches a size where nutrients cannot be obtained by simple diffusion. The tumor needs a blood supply. In a cell culture model where no blood supply exists, tumor spherules will grow to about 0.5 millimeter in maximum size. After that, new cell growth on the surface of the sphere is balanced by cell death from anoxia in the center. If cancers could only grow to a size smaller than a pinhead, they would be of almost no clinical significance. The process whereby a growing tumor recruits a new blood supply from the body is called **angiogenesis**. There is much debate as to what degree the tumor is responsible for recruiting growth of capillaries. The natural repair processes of the body supply new capillary growth in areas of tissue damage and inflammation. Some factors secreted by tumors act as growth factors on the surrounding normal tissue, invoking both the proliferation of fibroblasts and capillaries. If tumors had a specific angiogenic growth factor, then inhibition of this factor could be an important anticancer therapy (as will be discussed again in Chapter 11).

What is very clear is the realization that a growing tumor must overcome tissue barriers. Figure 5.3 shows schematically a small squamous cell carcinoma of the bronchus of the lung just beginning to invade deeper tissues. This small cancer has begun to recruit budding capillaries. The

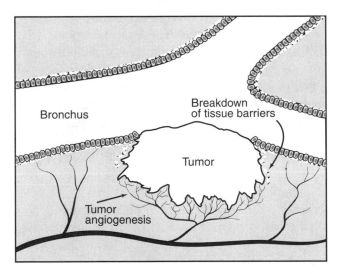

FIGURE 5.3. A tumor develops beyond microscopic size by the processes of angiogenesis and invasion through tissue barriers.

endothelial cells are proliferating in response to some local growth factor. An intense angiogenic stimulus is present, leading to multiple branching of the local vessels. We can envision that this 1-centimeter-diameter tumor as depicted with a very good blood supply will grow much faster than one with a limited blood supply.

Tissue Invasion and Metastasis

In addition to developing a blood supply, tumors must overcome tissue barriers in order to invade. The hallmark of cancer as recognized by the pathologist under the microscope is invasion through local tissue barriers. Most cancers have a recognizable **carcinoma *in-situ*** stage where the tumor is confined to the epithelial layer. Carcinoma *in situ* is likely curable by surgical excision. The goal of early clinical detection of cancer is to find tumors at this stage. Unfortunately, cancers are usually detected only at more advanced stages. About one-third of cancer patients present as advanced stage disease with distant clinical metastases. Another third present with locally invasive disease, but no clinical evidence of metastasis. Unfortunately, clinical experience demonstrates that for many forms of cancer such as lung, colon, breast, or prostate, there is a high probability that nondetected micrometastases are already present when the tumor is locally invasive. Only one third of patients are diagnosed with truly localized disease that is surgically resectable, with a low likelihood of metastasis.

The process of tissue invasion and metastasis is therefore very relevant in the clinical management of cancer. For most cancers derived from epithelium, such as colon, cervix, and breast (as we will discuss in Chapters 8, 9, and 10), we can identify patients at the clinical stage of carcinoma *in situ*. At this point, the tumor is a clonal malignancy. However, this clonal neoplasm has not extended beyond the retaining basement membrane that underlies all epithelium. The basement membrane is an extracellular structure made up of collagen (type IV), and glycoproteins including laminin and fibronectin. Epithelial cells have receptors for these molecules. The basement membrane provides a barrier and a point of anchorage for the epithelial cells. Normal cells cannot grow and function without this point of attachment. Cancer cells progressively lose this dependency on the basement membrane. In order to invade, the tumor must breach the basement membrane, usually by secreting collagenases and other enzymes that destroy connective tissue elements. These enzymes include plasminogen, cathepsins, and hyaluronidase. The invasion of the connective tissue by the tumor is a subversion of the body's normal inflammatory and repair processes.

At the next stage beyond carcinoma *in situ*, the tumor extends through the basement membrane. The enzymes that break down the local tissue barriers may serve as biomarkers of the tumor. Cathepsin D is a proteinase that is a marker of increased biological aggressiveness in breast cancer (see Chapter 10). Other biomarkers are related to surface molecules on cancer cells that correlate with their loss of dependence on attachment to the basement membrane. Like angiogenesis, tumor invasion through tissue barriers is a possible point at which to target new anticancer therapies. Some of the reported effects of drugs such as heparin and antiinflammatory agents on cancer may work at this stage.

After the tumor breaks through the basement membrane, the tumor cells invade the connective tissue. The tumor cells now have the potential to migrate into lymphatic or venous channels and propagate to distant parts of the body. To establish a metastasis, the tumor cells must survive the body's immune system. They must also find a tissue environment that will support their growth needs. Some tumors predictably metastasize to the most available downstream capillary bed. Breast cancer goes to lung; lung cancer goes to brain. Other tumor cells grow best in more specific environments. The bone marrow supplies a good microenvironment for metastasis. The characteristic special patterns of metastasis such as stomach cancer spreading to ovaries must indicate some hormonal or biochemical support of the tumor cells.

Tumor Immunology

Since tumors are derived from normal cells of the body, they are intrinsically recognized as "self" by the immune system. An important exception occurs when, as part of the cancer cell's abnormal function, it expresses an inappropriate antigen. How often does it happen that a cancer cell is recognized as foreign? The role of immune surveillance by the body as a means of keeping cancer in check has been debated for decades. Immune-compromised patients have a 10- to 20-fold increase in cancer, but this is due almost entirely to an increase in lymphomas. These lymphomas are likely due to mutations occurring in proliferating lymphocyte precursors not held in check by an intact immune system. The more common solid cancers are not increased in immune-compromised patients.* Thus, it is tempting to say that immune surveillance does not occur. That

---

*Squamous cell carcinoma of the cervix may be an exception (see Chapter 9). We are still learning a lot about cancer in immune-compromised patients.

conclusion is too limiting. Host immune reaction against tumor cells may be inconstant or ineffective, but it occurs. In Chapter 7, we will discuss the immune reaction that occurs when a leukemic patient undergoes bone marrow transplantation. The donor bone marrow reconstitutes a new immune system in the host. The reaction of the donor marrow graft against residual host leukemic cells is an important facet of the success of this therapy. Our ability to manipulate the immune system with genetically engineered lymphocytes, pharmed cytokines, and DNA vaccines may turn the limited response of the host into an effective anticancer therapy (see also Chapter 11).

What we would really like to identify in a cancer is a tumor specific antigen (TSA) not present on normal cells in the body. Even if the immune system does not respond strongly to a TSA, we can encourage it to do so. TSAs are rare in human tumors. A mutated cell only rarely produces a unique peptide that appears as an antigen to cytotoxic lymphocytes. More commonly tumors express "associated" antigens (TAA) that occur naturally on some normal cells. An example would be the expression of a fetal antigen on a pancreatic carcinoma cell. This antigen is derived from a gene that is normally silent in adult cells. The T-lymphocyte arm of the immune system may or may not react to the antigen, depending on whether it was conditioned to recognize the antigen as self during fetal development.

There is a great deal that we do not know about the immune system. I suspect we are not even halfway to a complete understanding. Lymphocytes do attack tumors, especially if given an extra stimulus to do so, even in the absence of a recognizable "nonself" marker. Natural killer (NK) lymphocytes bind to and lyse tumor cells by an unknown mechanism. Culturing a patient's lymphocytes with IL-2 cytokine and then reinfusing the lymphocytes sometimes produces a significant immune destruction of the tumor. This happens only some of the time. Similarly, macrophages may be stimulated to secrete tumor necrosis factor (TNF).

We will return to the problem of immune attack of tumors in Chapter 11 when we look at novel anticancer therapies in detail. The immune system's normal role in holding cancer in check is still very much in question.

The Complexity of the Immune System—An Aside

The complexity of the immune system is vastly underestimated; it rivals that of the central nervous system. Present the immune system with an antigen, and it might respond with anaphylaxis one time and the next time it might not respond at all. Tell a good joke, and your audience may convulse with laughter—or maybe not. Antigen response for the immune system or a laugh from the central nervous system depends on the situation. These systems are too complex to have a fixed "hard-wired" response.

The immune system has all the components necessary to be as sophisticated as the brain. (1) The immune system has memory. Immunoglobulin molecules are built to respond to antigens that are long gone. Memory lymphocytes have surface receptors to past stimuli. (2) The immune system has sensory input. Macrophages "taste" new objects and pass on what they have sensed. (3) The immune system has effector output. In response to stimuli it can release rapid or slow reactive substances like histamine and cytokines. (4) The immune system has processing. Antigen presenting cells like macrophages pass on their information to T lymphocytes. The interaction of the classes of T and B lymphocytes decides what response will be taken to the information. The information processing of the immune system is distributed rather than central. There is no spinal cord that can be cut that will stop everything. The immune system is distributed throughout the body. It communicates with its numerous cellular elements by molecular messengers and by direct cell-to-cell contact. (5) The immune system has programming. T lymphocytes are programmed, or "schooled," in the thymus. These five elements—memory, input, output, processing, and programming—constitute the organization of a complex system with the potential for actions that we cannot predict.

The basic blueprint of the immune system and of the brain is contained within the genome. But the details of the immune system and the brain are not. There are far more neuron-to-neuron connections in the nervous system than there are base pairs in the genome. The wiring pattern of the brain is not written in the genome. Neuron-to-neuron contacts develop according to algorithms and influences that we do not understand. The immune system is also a self-organizing system. The immune system like the brain builds itself based on what it experiences.

We know a few of the mechanisms for the building of the immune system. Immunoglobulin gene rearrangement permits a group of one hundred or so genes to be shuffled into coding for millions of antibodies. Repeat antigen stimulation produces an amplified secondary response in the number of clonal B lymphocytes synthesizing the corresponding antibody. The memory for the antigen is enhanced by repeated encounters. That is, unless the antigen is encountered too often, then the immune system becomes tolerant—like a too-often-repeated joke getting no response. Certain physiologic situations, like pregnancy, modulate the immune system. Drugs also nonspecifically blunt portions of the immune system.

Many aspects of the immune system are unknown, perhaps to a greater extent than we are aware. The most salient feature of the immune system is its ability to recognize self versus nonself. We do not understand fully how this comes about. Stem cells from umbilical cord blood may still be too naive to have this feature of the immune system "turned on." Cord blood stem cells may serve as a universal donor source for bone marrow transplantation. We can also transplant bone marrow between closely HLA matched siblings. If the match is good, the distinction between self and "sibling" is too fine to cause rejection by either side. The donor marrow takes several years to learn its new environment in the host. Only with significant time will the transplanted marrow ease its potential for graft versus host reactions. The transplanted marrow recapitulates early childhood development, relearning antigens. The immune system ages, losing function progressively after midlife. The thymus involutes; schooling of new T lymphocytes does not occur well after age 50. The immune system interacts with the other major organ systems. The central nervous system and the endocrine systems both influence and are influenced by the immune system. The best way to think about the immune system is to begin with a sense of wonder, and to realize that we have only begun to understand it.

Summary of Part I (Chapters 1–5)

Multiple Steps in Tumor Development

The development of cancer is a multistep process. Figure 5.4 demonstrates the first several steps in this process. The tumor begins at point (1) with an oncogene mutation in a single cell. The mutation results in a growth factor receptor with much greater than normal binding affinity. This cell, and all its progeny, will respond more rapidly to normal levels of growth factors than surrounding nonmutated cells. This growth advantage will lead to a slow clonal expansion of the mutated cell. We have, at this stage, a benign, well-differentiated tumor whose growth is still entirely dependent on external growth factor. A second mutation occurs at point (2) within one of the tumor cells in our original clone. This mutation is in the cell signal pathway, specifically in the K-ras oncogene. This oncogene protein affects the GTP and G protein related cell signal pathway. The mutated cell is now permanently stimulated independent of any external growth factor. This cell with two mutations undergoes rapid clonal expansion. The pressure of rapid growth causes more mutations to occur. Most of these mutations result in the death of the cell. The abnormal DNA is detected and the cell cycle checkpoint

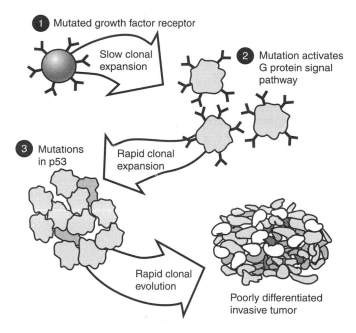

FIGURE 5.4. The progression of a neoplastic clone from benign to malignant demonstrates several successive mutations including: (1) a mutated growth factor receptor that confers a slight growth advantage; (2) a second mutation in the cell signal pathway that permits more rapid growth without external factors; and (3) loss of p53 tumor suppressor gene function. The end point is rapid growth and accumulation of more DNA errors resulting in a poorly differentiated invasive cancer

stops proliferation of the damaged cell. Unfortunately at point (3) a cell arises with both copies of its p53 tumor suppressor gene mutated. This cell is not subject to arrest at the cell cycle checkpoint. A very rapid growth of this new mutation occurs, with many further mutations developing because DNA repair and apoptosis are not functioning. We get rapid clonal evolution of the tumor, with the fastest growing and most invasive cells proliferating.

The schematic diagram of the multistep development of a tumor shown in Figure 5.4 is from the cellular point of view. Each mutational step is reflected in a change in the biological behavior of the cell clone. A different view is shown in Figure 5.5, in which tumor development is depicted as sequential processes. Carcinogenesis is the first step, where DNA damage occurs. Chemicals, radiation, or viruses are the causes of the DNA damage. Following DNA damage is DNA repair. If DNA repair is unsuccessful, then a mutation results. We are essentially interested only in mutations that occur in oncogenes or tumor suppressor genes leading to development of a neoplastic clone.

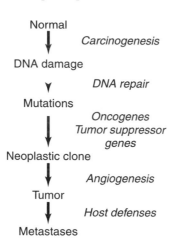

FIGURE 5.5. The evolution of a tumor can be seen as a series of processes.

The progression through the various steps shown in Figure 5.5 accelerates after oncogene and tumor suppressor gene mutation. The damage to the DNA has affected the cell's ability to repair itself, as well as deregulating cell proliferation. As the neoplastic clone grows beyond several millimeters in diameter, it must develop a blood supply. Tumor angiogenesis is an incompletely understood but necessary step for a clone to become a clinically significant tumor. Next the tumor begins its invasion of the body by overcoming host defenses. This includes the ability of the cancer cell to migrate through tissue barriers. The cancer cell must also evade the immune system. Finally, with host defenses defeated the tumor metastasizes and achieves its lethal potential.

Benign versus Malignant

At the molecular level, cancer is a multistep process. There is a continuum of change that occurs as a growth of cells develops from a slight disruption of normal to a poorly differentiated metastatic malignancy. Two cancers that clearly demonstrate this are adenocarcinoma of the colon (Chapter 8) and squamous cell carcinoma of the uterine cervix (Chapter 9). Both of these cancers develop slowly from well-recognized benign precursor lesions. We will discuss in those later chapters, the successive mo-lecular steps that occur as these cancers progress. What I hope to have already demonstrated, however, is that a tumor cannot be simply classified as either benign or malignant. The discovery of the molecular causes of cancer will require us to develop a more sophisticated classification of tumors. For example, a locally invasive ductal adenocarcinoma of the breast is unequivocally malignant. Yet additional molecular markers of the tumor such as DNA content, cell cycle proliferative index, and hormone receptors may demonstrate that this par-

*ticular malignant tumor has very likely not yet developed metastatic po-
tential and is curable by local excision (see Chapter 10). At this point
in our tour of molecular cancer medicine, we have seen enough of the
details of how DNA may be altered to understand that cancer is more
complex than an all or none phenomenon.*

References

Denissenko MF, Pao A, Tang M, et al. Preferential formation of benzo[a]pyrene
    adducts at lung cancer mutational hotspots in P53. *Science.* 1996;274:430–432.
Perera FP. Environment and cancer: who are susceptible? *Science.* 1997;278:
    1068–1073.
Ries LAG, Kosary CL, Hankey BF, Harras A, Miller BA, Edwards BK, eds.
    SEER Cancer Statistics Review, 1973-1993: Tables and Graphs. Bethesda:
    National Cancer Institute; 1996.

PART II

Clinical Examples
of Molecular Oncology

The second half of this book explores clinical examples that demonstrate the basic molecular biology of cancer and the role of oncogenes. I hope to prove to you that the basic science we learned in the first section is not purely theoretical. Basic science immediately leads to new diagnostic techniques and to new therapies. In fact, the second section begins with "Molecular Diagnostics" and concludes with "Molecular Anti-Cancer Therapies." In between, we look at four types of tumors: leukemia/lymphoma, colon cancer, squamous cell carcinoma of the cervix, and breast cancer. The central theme is DNA damage as it accumulates, leading through the multiple steps of cancer development. In chronic myeloid leukemia and Burkitt's lymphoma, we see in detail how a specific oncogene mutation results in cancer. For colon cancer, we see the progressive evolution from benign neoplastic polyp to atypical villous adenoma to invasive cancer with DNA changes occurring at each step. In the following chapter, we consider carcinoma of the cervix as a viral-induced cancer. Should it best be treated or prevented with a vaccine? The chapter on the molecular biology of breast cancer raises as-yet-unanswered questions. Molecular biology will show us why breast cancer is such a clinically complex disease with variable behavior from patient to patient.

This book is not a monograph reporting all that is currently known about the molecular biology of cancer. My goal is to increase our knowledge and understanding of the basic principles and to apply them to a few cancers. Keep in mind that much detail has been omitted to allow these basic principles to stand out clearly. Remember in addition that our knowledge of the molecular biology of cancers is growing rapidly. Each week some discovery reveals, amplifies, and corrects what we thought we knew the week before.

Molecular Diagnostics

Overview

Molecular diagnostics seeks to detect errors that cause disease at the level of DNA. This is a rapidly evolving field with new technologies leapfrogging over previous methods. Unthinkable only a few years ago, now the most direct method of examining DNA is sequencing by automated methods. This chapter discusses the clinical laboratory tools available and probable near future developments. Surprisingly, I think that I will soon make apparent to you that our molecular technology is already well developed. Where we are stuck is limited clinical experience. Molecular diagnostics can detect disease at a level that we are only now ready to address. The major breakthroughs in molecular diagnostics await physicians discovering the correct use of the technology.

Scale of Damage to DNA

The scale of damage to DNA that concerns us as we devise molecular diagnostic technologies is quite large. To look at a molecular abnormality in a colon polyp, we may want to detect a single point mutation, such as a change from A to G in codon 59 of the *ras* gene. An appropriate technique would be a gene probe. On the other hand, to assess the biological aggressiveness of a colon cancer we measure whether the tumor is aneuploid. This is a change of at least 100 million base pairs! The appropriate technique to measure aneuploidy is cytometry. Recall our library analogy of the information content of the human genome. A point mutation is a misspelling in a single word (codon), within a paragraph (exon), in one book (gene), located on one set of shelves (chromosome) in the library (genome). A gene probe looks for a misspelled word. The determination of aneuploidy by flow or image cytometry requires the explosive destruction of at least 10% of the entire library!

Table 6.1 lists examples that demonstrate the scale of DNA damage that we wish to detect in various molecular diagnostic problems. Let us consider the laboratory methods available to us, working from the top down. We will start with the detection of aneuploid DNA and abnormal cell cycle parameters by cytometry. Next, we will drop down to the level of the chromosome, looking at karyo-types and the modern technique of fluorescent *in situ* hybridization (FISH). Finally, we will consider the major gene probe methods: Southern blot, polymerase chain reaction (PCR), DNA on a chip, and genome sequencing.

Cytometry

Cytometry is the science of making measurements on individual cells. Not so long ago, we considered the cell to be the smallest unit for our examination. Now the cell is a virtual galaxy of molecules, interacting under the guidance of DNA at the center in the nucleus. However, the cell is still important! Cancer does not become a disease until damage to DNA permanently alters the behavior of a cell and all its progeny. We use cytometers to measure cells and check on their function.

There are two basic types of cytometers: flow and image. Both look at cells. In **flow cytometry**, cells are in a liquid suspension passing through an orifice one at a time. A laser beam probes the cell for size, internal structure, and the presence of fluorescent markers. In **image cytometry**, the cells are viewed on a glass slide through a conventional microscope.

Table 6.1. Scale of DNA damage in molecular diagnostics.

Base pairs affected	Appropriate technology	Clinical examples
$1-10^6$	Gene probes	
	Southern blot	Lymphoma, clonal population
	PCR	H-*ras* point mutation
	DNA on a chip	p53, large deletions
	Sequencing	*BRCA*1 mutations
	Protein truncation	Other *BRCA*1 mutations
10^6-10^8	Karyotype analysis, FISH	t(9;22) *BCR/ABL*
		t(15;17) *RARa/PML*
10^9	Cytometry, flow and image	Aneuploidy in colon, and breast carcinomas

A color digital camera and a computer measure cell features, particularly the density of marker stains. Both methods can measure the amount of DNA inside a cell. Flow cytometers measure the fluorescent signal from a DNA binding dye such as propidium iodide. Image cytometers measure the overall gray density of a DNA stain such as Feulgen in the nucleus. Flow cytometers typically look at 1000 cells per second; image cytometers look at one cell in about 15 seconds (or as fast as we can click on them—human decision limits the speed).

Cytograms

The DNA content of cells is usually reported as a cytogram, graphing the number of cells versus their relative DNA content. Figure 6.1 shows a flow cytogram of a breast carcinoma. There are two peaks. The left hand peak has a **DNA index** of 1.0 and represents normal breast epithelial cells with diploid DNA content. The second peak shifted to the right has a DNA index of 1.86 and represents an aneuploid population of malignant breast carcinoma cells. The mean DNA content of this population is 1.86 times the normal diploid DNA content. These cells have an extra 5 billion base pairs of DNA, or the equivalent of an extra 40 chromosomes! Not all breast cancers are aneuploid. The ploidy and cell cycle parame-

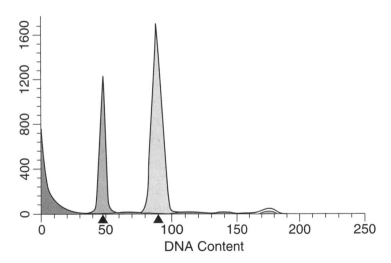

FIGURE 6.1. Flow cytogram of DNA ploidy in a biopsy sample of invasive ductal carcinoma of the breast. Two populations are seen, the left hand peak (25%) representing diploid cells and the right hand peak (75%) representing aneuploid tumor cells with a ploidy index of 1.86.

ters determined by flow cytometry of this patient's tumor suggest increased biological aggressiveness, as will be discussed in Chapter 10.

Figure 6.2 is an image cytogram of a prostate carcinoma, measured on a slide prepared as part of routine processing of a needle biopsy of a prostate nodule. Figure 6.3 is a picture of what the image cytometer "sees" in making this analysis. Each nucleus is an array of dots of varying gray scales. The integration of these gray scales determines the amount of DNA in that nucleus. The image cytogram in Figure 6.2 shows a population of aneuploid prostate adenocarcinoma cells. The mean DNA content of the cancer cells is a DNA index of 1.42 or 10.1 picograms of DNA per cell. The image cytogram in Figure 6.2 is much less smooth than the flow cytogram in Figure 6.1. This is because only 150 cells were measured in the image analysis versus 20,000 cells in the flow analysis.

The analysis of the DNA content of a population of cells detects the ploidy and the distribution of the population through the G1, S, and G2 compartments of the cell division cycle. Review Figure 2.1. Tumor populations with more than 5% to 10% cells within the S phase of the cell cycle are rapidly dividing. Flow cytometry produces a precise measure of the S phase fraction because of the large number of cells analyzed. In the cytogram shown in Figure 6.1 of a breast carcinoma, computer analysis of the two populations gives us an S phase of 13% for the diploid and 9% for the aneuploid. The S phase fraction of the tumor population is another parameter in addition to aneuploidy that indicates the biological aggressiveness for this patient's tumor. In this case, the S phase fraction of the aneuploid cells is slightly elevated.

The image cytogram of a prostate adenocarcinoma shown in Figure 6.2 is based on too few cells to get more than a qualitative estimate of the S phase fraction. In this case, we can only add the comment that the S phase fraction appears low. Image cytometry is best utilized for sampling small populations of tumor cells that infiltrate normal tissues. In the image cytometer, the operator can look at each cell under the microscope and choose which to analyze. In flow cytometry, all cells of a certain size or other defining characteristic are analyzed. Table 6.2 compares the features of image and flow cytometry for the analysis of ploidy and S phase fraction in tumors, showing the relative advantages of each.

Clinical Utility

Cytometry has been an available clinical laboratory method for tumor analysis for more than 10 years. We are still learning how to use the data to refine the diagnosis, treatment choices, and prognosis for individual patients. Table 6.3 lists some of the cancers in which cytometry has been

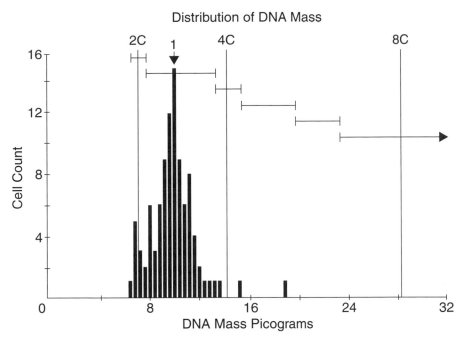

FIGURE 6.2. Image cytogram of aneuploidy in adenocarcinoma of the prostate. The distribution of DNA mass of the nuclei for 150 cells shows a broad peak around a mean of 10.1 picograms.

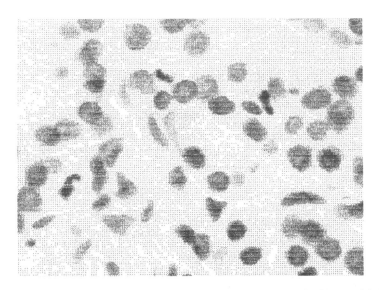

FIGURE 6.3. Pixel image of biopsy slide from case shown in Figure 6.2. The image is a series of gray dots, each representing the amount of DNA staining at that point.

Table 6.2. Flow versus image cytometry.

	Flow	Image
Number of cells analyzed	10^4	10^2
Rate of analysis	10^3/sec	10^{-1}/sec
Ploidy	High precision	Adequate precision
S phase, %	Quantitative	Qualitative
Sample type	Cell suspension	Biopsy on a slide cytology smears
Sample discrimination	Gating on size, or surface marker	Operator chooses cells individually

generally agreed to supply useful additional parameters for the staging or management of patients. For some tumors, the most important parameter is ploidy. For other cancers, the S phase is more important. Ploidy is a coarse measurement of the accumulation of a lot of DNA damage. An aneuploid cell has many mutations. The aneuploid malignant tumor cell is the endpoint of multistep tumor development, shown as step 4 in Figure 5.5. Cells with a high S phase fraction are rapidly dividing, which implies limited G1 checkpoint control. Rapidly dividing tumors, however, are amenable to some types of chemotherapy. Cytometry lets us measure the latter stages of progression in multistep cancer development. Cytometry adds additional staging parameters that individualize the prediction of how a patient's tumor might behave. A colon cancer that is diploid is of lower biological aggressiveness than one that is aneuploid.

I must admit that Table 6.3 would engender much debate among peo-

Table 6.3. Clinical utility of flow and image cytometry.

Tumor	Ploidy	S phase fraction	Preferred method*
Breast cancer	+/?	+	Flow
Colon cancer	+	+	Flow
Colon polyp	−/?	. . .	Flow
Endometrial cancer	+	?	Flow
Esophagus, Barrett's	+/?	. . .	Image
Leukemia/lymphoma	−	−	Flow
Ovarian cancer	+/?	+/?	Flow
Prostate cancer	+/?	?	Image/flow
Renal cancer	+/?	?	Flow
Urinary bladder transitional cell	+	?	Image/flow

*The preferred method depends on the type of sample available. Needle biopsies with a small amount of tumor and many cytology preparations can be done only by image.

ple who use cytometry data. There is still no solid consensus on which patients should have cytometry testing done even after a decade of experience. Breast, colon, prostate, ovary, and endometrial carcinomas are those most commonly studied by cytometry for the additional prognostic information these results supply. Like some of our other molecular diagnostic tests, the big question remains, "What can I do with this information to help my patient?"

Chromosome Analysis

Karyotype

Anyone who has watched a living cell divide under a microscope cannot help but be fascinated with the movement of the chromosomes. Chromosomes just look important, and they are! Recall Figure 1.1 and reflect on the complex spiral organization of the DNA strand around the nucleosomes as they pack into a chromosome. Very careful technique allows some of this complex structure to be visualized, permitting chromosome analysis or **karyotype**. A karyotype is constructed by culturing cells, harvesting them at the midpoint of mitosis, and smearing the chromosomes on a glass slide. The technique for spreading the chromosomes is important. You want to have them really squashed, but not broken, so that you can see the details. The method I was taught is to hold a pipette containing the cell suspension out in front of my chin and drip them onto a glass slide on the floor. The slide is tilted at a 45° angle to let the drop hit hard and then slide. The whole affair looks like an Olympic ski jump. After a few drops have successfully hit their target, the slide is carefully stained with Giemsa dye that reveals bands on the chromosomes related to different densities of DNA and protein. If the technique sounds finicky, that's the point. Karyotyping cells for many years was an art form as well as a science. A lot of differences that caused arguments were due to technique. Now karyotyping, although still requiring careful methodology, is a standardized procedure giving important details of genomic damage at the large scale of the chromosome.

Figure 6.4 is a karyotype of a leukemic cell from a patient with chronic myeloid leukemia (CML). The chromosomes have been stained with Giemsa dye that reveals a pattern of bands. The physical location of a gene on a chromosome is defined according to these bands. The long arm of a chromosome is designated q, the short arm p. Regions on each arm are numbered according to major and minor bands. In CML, a translocation between the long arms of chromosomes 9 and 22 occurs. Both the abnormal chromosomes 9 and 22 are marked with arrows in the figure.

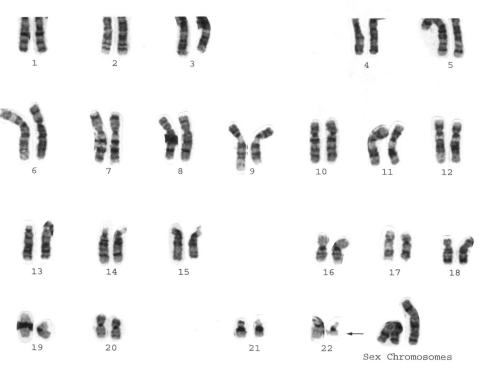

FIGURE 6.4. Karyotype analysis of a cell from a patient with chronic myeloid leukemia demonstrating a reciprocal translocation between the long arms of chromosomes 9 and 22 (arrows). The short abnormal "Philadelphia" chromosome 22 was the first clonal marked discovered in a malignancy. This karyotype provided by Mark Pettenati of Wake Forest University School of Medicine.

The short chromosome 22, denoted t(9;22)q34q11, is seen only in CML. Initially described by Peter Nowell in Philadelphia, the Philadelphia chromosome was the first clonal abnormality discovered in a malignancy.

Fluorescent *In Situ* Hybridization (FISH)

The visualization of chromosomes has recently been greatly aided by combining karyotype and gene probes. This process is called **FISH** (fluorescent *in situ* hybridization). The Giemsa banded chromosomes demonstrated in Figure 6.4 only occur when the genetic material of the cell is organized as a metaphase chromosome during mitosis. This happens very rarely in the natural life of a cell. Chromosomes are not recognizable in a cell by karyotype analysis except at mitosis. The use of probes that bind to specific base pair sequences unique to each chromosome has extended our ability to "watch" the chromosomes. The probes used in the FISH technique carry a chemical tag that makes them visible in a fluorescent microscope. Multiple probes can be used, each with a different color.

Figure 6.5 shows a photograph of two interphase (or nonmitotic) cell nuclei probed for the *ABL* oncogene on chromosome 9 and the *BCR* gene on chromosome 22. These two cells are also from a CML patient. The first cell (A) is normal. The open arrowheads indicate two separate *ABL* signals (which appear red on the color version of this photograph). Two closed arrowheads indicate separate *BCR* signals (green). This cell does

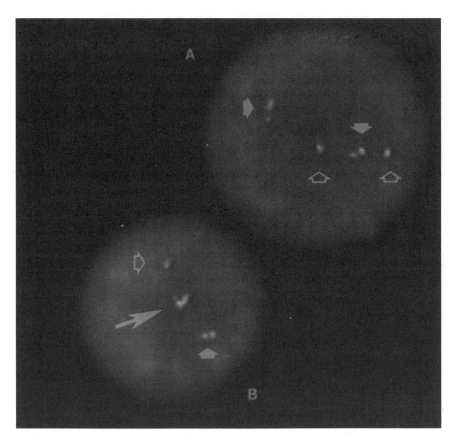

FIGURE 6.5. FISH chromosome analysis of two cells from a patient with chronic myeloid leukemia. Cell A is normal and shows two *ABL* signals (open arrowheads) and two *BCR* signals (closed arrowheads). Cell B shows one normal *ABL* and *BCR* signal, as well as a fused signal with *BCR* and *ABL* touching (large arrow). In the original color fluorescent photograph the *ABL* signal is red and the *BCR* signal green. The FISH analysis provided by Mark Pettenati of Wake Forest University School of Medicine.

not show a translocation fusing these two genes, i.e., the Philadelphia chromosome is not present. The second cell (B) is abnormal demonstrating one *ABL* (open arrowhead) and one *BCR* (closed arrowhead) signal along with a fused signal (large arrow). In the color version of this photograph the two dots at the end of the long arrow are red and green. From the data in this photograph, we can conclude that cell (B) has one t(9;22) Philadelphia chromosome.

In the FISH technique, we can analyze several chromosomes, even though the cell is not in mitosis! FISH is a significant advance in chromosome analysis because most cancer cells cannot be studied by the standard karyotype technique. We are no longer limited to looking at only those cells that we can grow in culture and artificially stimulate into mitosis. We will discuss the molecular biology of CML in detail in Chapter 7. We now understand how the fusion of the *ABL* and *BCR* genes causes the abnormal proliferation of the leukemic cells.

The FISH technique can look at several chromosomes simultaneously, or one chromosome in greater detail. The hybridization of probes to chromosomes greatly helps in producing a physical map for the human genome, and allows for detail analysis of physical changes in the genome. Mark Pettenati of Wake Forest University provided these two excellent photos (Figures 6.4 and 6.5). Cytogenetics is very technical, and requires experience provided by Mark in how to interpret the data. This is a theme that we will see over and over with new molecular diagnostic techniques.

FISH is an easier and more generally applicable technique than Giemsa banded karyotype analysis when looking for a specific abnormal chromosome. FISH can be applied to cell imprints from tumors, cell suspensions, and many other clinical samples. For example, a glass slide touched to the fresh cut surface of a biopsy of a colon tumor provides an imprint suitable for FISH. FISH is an illustrative and analytic bridge between genomic probes and looking at entire chromosomes.

Combining karyotype and FISH, a number of nonrandom chromosome events have been detected in a wide variety of cancers. I say nonrandom chromosome events because many, if not most, cancer cells have a background of random broken chromosomes. Every aneuploid cancer cell has some broken, deleted, or duplicated chromosomes. However, each cell is different in the fragments detected. We are interested only in repetitive identical abnormal chromosomes that can be seen in every cell. These nonrandom chromosome events mark a clone and possibly point to the early genetic events for that tumor. A rough analogy would be to compare the cytogeneticist to a fire marshal. The problem is to probe through the wreckage of a fire gutted home in order to find the electrical short in a light bulb on the Christmas tree that caused the fire. Fortunately, like the fire marshal, the cytogeneticist has developed the experience of where to look. Table 6.4 lists a few examples of abnormal chromosomes associated with various tumors. I have also listed the oncogene or tumor suppressor genes that are implicated at the site of chromosome damage. Leukemia and lymphoma appear more commonly than other cancers in this table. This is because leukemia cells are more easily sampled, even repeatedly, from a patient than cells from solid cancers like lung and colon. Leukemia and lymphoma cells are more easily cultured, and therefore subjects for karyotype analysis. FISH and other molecular probes will allow Table 6.4 to be greatly expanded to other tumors.

Gene Probes

Southern Blot

The Southern blot was one of the methods that constituted the revolution called "recombinant DNA technology." Prior to about 1975, the only way to probe the genome of an organism was to do breeding experiments!

Table 6.4. Nonrandom chromosome events in cancer—selected examples.

Tumor	Chromosome event	Oncogene tumor suppressor gene
Carcinoma		
Breast carcinoma	del(1p)	?
Lung carcinoma		
Small cell	del(3)	?
Large cell	del(9)	?
Renal carcinoma	del(3)	?*VHL*
Sarcoma		
Ewing's sarcoma/PNET/Askin tumor	t(11;22)	*EWS*
Liposarcoma	t(12;16)	?
Melanoma	del(1) del(6)	?
Leukemia/lymphoma		
Chronic myeloid leukemia	t(9;22)	*BCR/ABL*
Acute promyelocytic leukemia	t(15;17)	*PML/RAR*
Burkitt's lymphoma	t(8;14)	*myc*
Follicular lymphoma	t(14;18)	bcl-2
Mantle cell lymphoma	t(11;14)	CYCLIN D1

Genetics up to that time was in the era of the fruit fly, yeast, bacteria, and viruses. The small amount known about the human genome prior to 1975 was learned from genetic diseases. The best known human genes in terms of large-scale population data were those of the blood group antigens. Some geneticists were so pessimistic about the possibility of ever understanding the immensity of the human genome that they considered the subject a dead end. The Southern blot with restriction enzymes was the method that began the current era.

The **Southern blot** is named after its inventor, Ed Southern. The blot is a method for analyzing DNA by: (1) cutting DNA into pieces with a restriction enzyme; (2) electrophoresing the pieces to separate them according to size; and (3) probing by hybridization to identify a single DNA segment of interest. The same procedure applied to RNA is called a **Northern blot**, and when applied to protein a **Western blot**. These names are a joke on Ed Southern's name and a tribute to him. We will briefly consider each step in the process.

Restriction Enzymes

A restriction endonuclease (enzyme) is a protein derived from bacteria that cuts DNA at a specific nucleotide sequence. The **restriction enzyme Bgl II*** cuts DNA wherever it encounters the base pair sequence AGATCT. The cut is made between the first A and the following G. These six nucleotides occur at approximately 20,000 sites over the 6,000,000,000 bp of the human genome. If you incubate a solution of DNA with Bgl II at 37°C for 30 minutes, you will have cut the human genome into 20,000 fragments from about 5 to 20 kb each. DNA extracted from human cells before cutting exists as a few very large strands approaching hundreds of millions of base pairs in length. Since DNA of this size breaks so easily with simple stirring of the test tube, no one is sure of the original "native" length of the DNA molecules in our cells.

Hundreds of restriction enzymes are now in use for the purpose of cutting DNA into manageable and reproducible fragments. Restriction enzymes exist in bacteria for the purpose of protecting them from bacterio-

---

*Bgl II is pronounced "bagel two." Recombinant DNA technology is full of jargon, nonstandard abbreviations, and local lab customs. The spirit that existed in the early DNA labs, and to a degree continues to this day, is a surprising blend of high science and cult. The hot-shot graduate students who mastered a new technique invented their own words and style. A reliable restriction enzyme is called a *good cutter* because, like a comfortable pair of scissors, it does its job.

phage. Restriction enzymes constitute a primitive immune system for bacteria. When the genetic material of a bacteriophage enters a bacterium, the phage's genome is cut if it contains the specific sequences recognized by the bacterium's restriction enzyme. The restriction enzymes have evolved to recognize sequences that occur in the invading phage, but do not occur in the bacterial genome. This type of immune system fails in higher organisms with larger genomes. It is not possible to write very long genetic messages without using the five or six letter combinations that restriction enzymes recognize. Restriction enzymes, besides serving bacteria as an immune system, are a fundamental tool allowing us to cut DNA at a specific site. This cutting is used in the Southern blot analysis, as well as in cloning, and almost all other recombinant DNA techniques.

Hybridization Probes

Our ability to probe the human genome is based upon the affinity for complementary base sequences to recognize each other and to form a reversible chemical bond. To find a specific gene, we make a probe that is complementary. The probe needs to be labeled in some way, with a colored, or luminescent, or radioactive tag attached to the nucleic acid. We then incubate our DNA sample with the probe under conditions that permit the **hybridization** or bonding of the probe to the target. These conditions include choosing the temperature, pH, and salt concentration. By slightly altering the conditions we can require an exact match between our probe and target, or just an approximate match. Varying the conditions is called choosing the stringency of the hybridization. At the end of the incubation, we look for our tag and that shows us where the target is. In the Southern blot method, our hybridization is performed on a membrane that has been blotted against the DNA electrophoresis gel. The single fragment that contains our target sequence shows up as a colored band on the blot. Figure 6.6 is a Southern blot analysis of the T-lymphocyte receptor gene. The bands are shown for the native or germline configuration of the gene, as well as for a clonal rearrangement that indicates a T-cell lymphoma, as will be discussed in Chapter 7.

Let's look at another example of hybridization using a short synthetic probe for the c-*myc* oncogene. Listed below is a nucleotide sequence that occurs at the start of the amino acid coding portion of the second exon of the c-*myc* oncogene. In italics I have repeated its complementary form:

. . . ATGCCCCTCAACGTTAGCTTC . . .

TACGGGGAGTTGCAATCGAAG

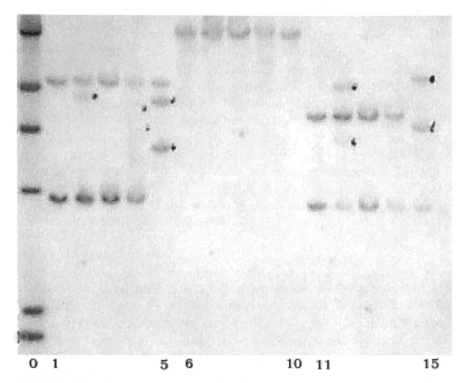

FIGURE 6.6. A Southern blot analysis of the T-cell receptor gene shows re-arranged bands (marked with dots) in several DNA samples from patients.

The 21 base pairs beginning ATG . . . do not occur in this order at any other point in the genome. We can synthesize the short piece of complementary DNA shown in italics. This is easy to do in an automated machine. A number of services are listed in the back of all the molecular biology journals that offer overnight delivery of synthetic oligomers, currently for about $1 per nucleotide. We may choose to order our 21 bp oligonucleotide piece (also called a 21mer) already labeled, or maybe we will put on the label ourselves.

The c-*myc* oncogene is translocated in Burkitt's lymphoma from its normal location on chromosome 8 to a site adjacent to the immunoglobulin heavy chain gene on chromosome 14, a t(8;14) lesion. We can use our 21mer c-*myc* probe to detect this translocation on a Southern blot. Moving the gene changes the pattern of fragments when the gene is digested with restriction enzymes.

But we can do a lot more than just diagnose the molecular lesion of Burkitt's lymphoma. If we want to observe whether a particular course of chemotherapy is affecting the tumor, we might want to look at the *expression* of c-*myc* in the tumor cells. We can do this with a Northern blot, looking for the presence or absence of c-*myc* messenger RNA (mRNA). The presence of mRNA indicates the gene is "turned on" (i.e., being expressed). You will recall from Chapter 3 that c-*myc* expression is a stimulus for the tumor cells to divide.

Going one step further, we can use hybridization to block c-*myc* gene expression. Now our probe becomes therapy! A piece of DNA that is complementary to c-*myc* mRNA is called an **antisense oligonucleotide**. This is because its DNA sequence is in the inverted complementary sense to that of the mRNA strand. If we can get the antisense molecule into the tumor cells, it will hybridize to the c-*myc* mRNA strand. This prevents the strand from being read into a protein by the cell's polyribosomes. This is called *antisense therapy*, and we will talk more about it in coming chapters, especially Chapter 11. All of these tools are derived from the basic principle of complementary base pair sequence hybridizing.

Polymerase Chain Reaction (PCR)

The Southern blot method lasted for a little more than a decade as the major gene analysis tool. Now the polymerase chain reaction (**PCR**) has virtually replaced it. I will describe PCR briefly. I warn you that most people need it explained two or three times before they get it. That's not because it is difficult, it's so simple! The story by Kary Mullis of his invention of PCR in 1984 is fascinating (Mullis, 1994) and I recommend it to you. PCR is an amplification technology. The sought after DNA target sequence is detected by making millions of copies of it, so it is easy to see against the background of all the other DNA fragments. The PCR technique like most molecular technologies is based on hybridization.

A DNA mix is hybridized with two short DNA probes called amplimers (for amplification oligonucleotides). The amplimers bind on either side of the target DNA sequence. One amplimer binds on one of the two DNA strands; the other amplimer binds to the opposite strand. When double-stranded DNA is heated to near 100°C, it melts into two single strands. The reaction mixture is then cooled to about 60°C. The short amplimers hybridize to the target site on the single-stranded DNA. An enzyme called **DNA polymerase** begins making new double-stranded DNA. The DNA polymerase requires a short double-stranded region of DNA to prime its copying function. New double-stranded DNA is synthesized only at the locations where the amplimers have hybridized to the target. These sites are the only double-stranded regions in our test tube. The new double-strand DNA synthesis extends along the DNA strand, heading from the 5' end towards 3', at about 1000 bp per second under the action of the DNA polymerase. This extension is usually done at a slightly higher temperature, about 72°C. After a short while we have *two double-strand* copies of our target DNA. We heat the test tube back up to 95°C, and the DNA again melts. Now we have *four single* strands of our target to which the amplimers can bind. We cool back down to 60°, rehybridize the amplimers, and then warm to 72° to extend. Bang! In a few minutes we have eight strands of target DNA. Every time we cycle between 60, 72, and 95°C, we double the number of copies of our target DNA.

A PCR reaction usually involves 30 cycles and takes 4 hours. The reaction is carried out in a small box called a thermal cycler that holds 100-uL test tubes in a metal block. The metal changes temperatures quickly under computer control. The real neat thing about PCR was finding a DNA polymerase that did not mind being exposed to temperatures near boiling! Almost all enzymes work best at 37°C and are denatured into an inactive form by boiling. That's why cooking works. However, very smart people realized that the algae living in the hot geysers in Yellowstone National Park must have a DNA polymerase happy at near boiling temperatures. The enzyme cloned from these algae is called **Taq** (for *Thermal aquaticus*, the name of the algae).

As we will see in later sections, PCR can detect specific genome sequences with great sensitivity and specificity. For example, in Chapter 7 we will see that CML is caused by abnormal fusion gene, *BCR/ABL*. The PCR method can detect this gene sequence, even when only a few leukemic cells are present. PCR is also very good at detecting viruses and determining whether the viral genome has been inserted into the cellular DNA.

DNA on a Chip

The scale and density of information stored in DNA begs for analogies. One has been to compare DNA to microcomputer chips. The idea is valid, although DNA stores information on a much smaller physical scale. A single base pair occupies 3.4×10^{-9} meters along the DNA helix and the whole genome weighs only 7×10^{-12} grams (from Table 1.1). A more useful aspect of the DNA to computer chip analogy is the realization that the micro-tools of semiconductor technology can lead to the design of automated, efficient molecular diagnostics.

One approach (Affymetrix, Santa Clara, Ca; Fodor, 1997) uses light to direct the synthesis of small fragments of DNA on a semiconductor chip.

On a silicon substrate 10 millimeters across, an array of 32 by 32 individual sites is established. At each site, one nucleotide at a time, specific oligonucleotide probes are built up by combinatorial chemical synthesis. Photomasking allows each of the 1024 sites on the chip to be addressed uniquely as chemical synthesis proceeds. This is similar to the complex multilayering construction of very large scale integrated circuit (VLSI) microprocessors. The result is DNA on a chip, specifically 1024 distinct oligonucleotide probes. Much higher densities are possible.

The DNA chip is now ready to probe a test solution. The sample is first treated with enzymes to break down the tissue and release target DNA. This target DNA is then tagged with a fluorescent marker that will serve as a signal after hybridization. A tightly controlled mix of electrolytes and temperature is necessary to promote DNA hybridization between the target and the probes on the chip. The chip is immersed into the test solution. DNA binding between the sample and the probes (hybridization) occurs within seconds. Hybridization only occurs if a fragment in the test sample DNA is complementary to one of the probes on the chip. The 1024 different DNA probes on the chip allow analysis of multiple genes or gene sequencing.

After hybridization occurs during immersion in the test solution, the chip is then "read." A scanning laser confocal fluorescent microscope looks at each site on the chip. The confocal aspect of the microscope detects fluorescence bound to the surface plane of the chip. Only the surface of the chip is in focus. Unbound fluorescent sample DNA molecules floating in solution are out of the plane of focus and ignored. Automated scanning by the microscope produces an image of the entire surface of the chip in a few minutes. The sensitivity of the fluorescent microscope combined with optical amplifiers and image analysis is sufficient to detect only a few molecules of test DNA binding at any one of the sites on the chip. Current diagnostic applications of Affymetrix DNA chips include HIV sequencing and cystic fibrosis and *BRCA*1 mutation analysis. DNA on a chip has the ability to analyze simultaneously for the presence of hundreds of mutations. This makes cancer screening, such as *BRCA*1 testing, more feasible.

Other microtechnology approaches to molecular diagnosis are being examined. Again, the key has been to use the experience of the semiconductor industry to fabricate complex structures on a chip. One idea has been to fabricate an entire molecular laboratory as a microdevice. They propose putting PCR along with all the other steps of sample preparation and signal detection on a small semiconductor "chip." A stream of liquid containing the sample wends its way through channels only tens of microns in diameter, encountering the necessary reagents and conditions for PCR.

Another technology uses the principle of the ink jet printer, automating and miniaturizing the pipetting and sample preparation of a DNA lab.

Direct DNA Sequencing

As our ability to automate DNA analysis increases, we approach the point, unimaginable only a short while ago, of direct DNA sequencing. With automated instrumentation, it is possible to sequence a large gene within a day. For example, we can consider sequencing the entire *BRCA1* gene in a patient with a family history of breast cancer, not as research, but as a diagnostic test. The goal of the human genome project is to sequence the human genome once. Even before this great project is completed, the technology will have progressed to the point where single genes in patients can be sequenced on a routine basis. Over the last ten years, in terms of DNA analysis, it is as if we have progressed from the level of the Pony Express to a global satellite cellular phone system.

The techniques for direct DNA sequencing are all of the various gene probe technologies that we have so far considered, plus some new ones. The lesson for us is that as we discover genetic lesions diagnostic for cancer, we have the technology to find those lesions in patients.

Summary

Molecular diagnostics is adaptation of DNA technology for the purpose of detecting disease as it is expressed at the molecular level. Cancer is a multistep process caused by progressive damage to DNA. Molecular diagnostics allows us to measure this damage. A number of different techniques are available for looking at DNA, from large-scale damage at the level of multiple abnormal fragmented chromosomes (aneuploidy) down to single base pair mutations. We can look at populations of cells with flow and image cytometry; focus on single chromosomes by karyotype or FISH analysis; or analyze pieces of genes with Southern blot, PCR, and direct sequencing.

Our ability to examine DNA far outstrips our clinical experience. For a while we will be observing cancer at the molecular level, but uncertain as to how best to use the data. We have the opportunity to screen healthy people for inherited defects in tumor suppressor genes that predispose them to certain tumors. We will need to learn what to do with individuals discovered to be at great risk. We can study a colon polyp to see how far it has progressed in its evolution towards cancer. Will this affect our planned therapy?

References

Fodor SPA. Massively parallel genomics. *Science*. 1997;277:393–395.

Hannan RE. Future practices in diagnostic medicine. *Arch Pathol Lab Med* 1995;119:890–893.

Hess JL. Detection of chromosomal translocations in leukemia. Is there a best way? *Am J Clin Pathol*. 1998;109:3–5

Lipshutz RJ, Morris D, Chee M, Hubbell E, Kozal MJ, Shah N, Shen N, Yang R, Fodor SPA. Using oligonucleotide probe arrays to access genetic diversity. *Biotechniques*. 1995;19:442–447.

Ross DW. Clinical usefulness of DNA ploidy and cell cycle studies. *Arch Pathol Lab Med* 1993;117:1077.

Sinclair PB, Green AR, Grace C, Nacheva EP. Improved sensitivity of BCR-ADL detection: a triple-probe three-color fluorescence in situ hybridization system. *Blood*. 1997;90:1395–1402.

Leukemia and Lymphoma

Overview

The study of leukemia and lymphoma have always led the way in our understanding of the cellular and now the molecular biology of cancer. Leukemia and lymphoma cells are more readily accessible than are solid tumors. The malignant cells, when present in the blood, can be sampled daily. The Philadelphia chromosome that defines chronic myeloid leukemia (CML) was the first clonal marker discovered in a malignancy (Nowell, 1960). The molecular events underlying the Philadelphia chromosome translocation were one of the first discoveries of a translocated oncogene in human cancer (Groffen et al., 1984).

In this chapter we discuss four examples of malignancies, all characterized by a translocation of an oncogene or tumor suppressor gene. The translocation causes a mutation that leads to a clonal proliferation of cells resulting in a tumor. In the first example, CML, the translocation of the ABL *oncogene is sufficient to start the disease producing the chronic phase. Other mutations are necessary to spark chronic phase into an acute or blastic leukemia. The three lymphoma examples each demonstrate a different clinical course. The nature of lymphoma seems to depend on the "virulence" of the translocated gene.*

Molecular Evolution of a Leukemia

Case Presentation: Blast Crisis of Chronic Myeloid Leukemia

A 23-year-old male presented to the emergency department in a coma. His mother described 2 to 4 days of progressive weakness in her son. The patient had worked until 2 days before at his job as a roofing contractor. Physical exam showed an acutely ill, pale young male with shallow, rapid respirations and depressed mental status, responsive only to painful stimuli. The white blood cell count was 210,000/μl with a hemoglobin of 7.1

fusion gene that may affect the duration of chronic phase. The fact that chronic phase is extremely variable, lasting from months to decades, emphatically demonstrates that something must affect the pace of the disease. The only other fact that we know about our patient is that he had radiation exposure at age 5. A bad fracture of the foot was manipulated several times under fluoroscopic exam. Did x-rays at age 5 create double-strand breaks in a bone marrow stem cell later destined to become leukemic?

The purpose of this case example and the highly speculative time course that I have drawn in Figure 7.1 is to raise questions. At what point within this patient's 23 years would we, molecular doctors, say that this person "caught" leukemia? When could we best have taken preventative steps? When would we have wanted to start therapy? Let's examine the molecular biology of CML in more detail to see if we can answer, at least in part, these questions.

BCR/ABL Fusion Gene

The hallmark event of CML is the clonal marker first recognized as the Philadelphia chromosome t(9;22), and later characterized at the molecular level as a fusion between the *ABL* oncogene on chromosome 9 and the *BCR* gene on chromosome 22. *BCR/ABL* is seen in all CML patients.* The Philadelphia chromosome has occasionally been detected in patients several months prior to clinically apparent leukemia. It is not seen as an inherited chromosome defect, and the Philadelphia chromosome appears only in cell types derived from a pluripotent bone marrow stem cell (granulocytes, erythrocytes, megakaryocytes, monocyte/macrophages, and lymphocytes). Skin fibroblasts, buccal mucosa smears, or any other source of nonhematopoietic cells are Philadelphia negative in CML patients.

The *BCR/ABL* fusion gene is more than a marker of CML; there is sufficient molecular evidence to state that it causes the disease. The *ABL* proto-oncogene on chromosome 9 has two alternate first exons, 1a and 1b. In the normal expression of *ABL*, only one of these alternate exons is spliced to the downstream exons 2 through 11. There is a **splice acceptor site** in front of exon 2, and therein seems to lie the problem. This

---

*This is because I (and many, but not all of my colleagues) define CML by this molecular event. In a patient with a clinical syndrome resembling CML but lacking *BCR/ABL* fusion, I classify the patient as atypical CML. This is an important point. In the past, we have used morphology to classify diseases. Genetic lesions may be a more specific basis for defining disease.

splice acceptor site is "promiscuous" in that it accepts donors other than the expected upstream exon 1a or 1b. For reasons that still elude us, a portion of *BCR* on chromosome 22 can be matched to this site. Figure 7.2 shows a schematic map of *ABL, BCR,* and the abnormal *BCR/ABL* gene found only in CML patients.

I would like to speculate that some damage to the DNA on chromosomes 9 or 22 predisposes to the t(9;22) event. Perhaps an incorrectly repaired double-strand break or a carcinogen binding to the long stretch between exon 1a and 1b of *ABL* makes this happen. This speculation however has not been demonstrated experimentally. Whatever the cause, when *BCR/ABL* fuses, an activated oncogene is created. The protein product of *BCR/ABL* is a tyrosine kinase of molecular weight 210 kd. This tyrosine kinase has potent activity similar to that of the viral form of the abelson gene v-*ABL*. The exact mechanism by which *BCR/ABL* induces an expansion of the leukemic clone is unknown. However when the *BCR/ABL* gene is transfected into mice, a leukemia similar to the human disease results. There is even evidence that *BCR/ABL* can transfect cells in humans. In a few well documented cases, CML patients have been treated by bone marrow transplantation from a donor of the opposite sex. After transplant these patients have a reconstituted marrow showing the karyotype of the donor. Some patients have relapsed in the *donor* cells showing a *BCR/ABL* fusion gene that was identical to their original Philadelphia chromosome.

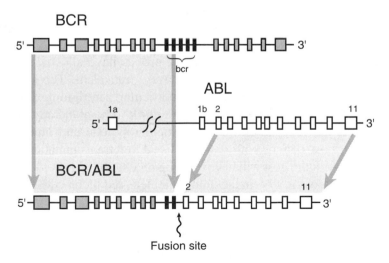

FIGURE 7.2. A gene map of *BCR/ABL* fusion shows that most of the *ABL* exons are carried over from chromosome 9 to 22.

The *BCR/ABL* fusion protein is a hyperactive tyrosine kinase. In Chapter 2 we demonstrated that proto-oncogenes code for steps in the cell signal pathway. A mutation of a proto-oncogene leads to an activated oncogene. This causes distortion of the signals that the cell receives and results in a clone of proliferating cells. *CML is an example of a cancer that develops because of a mutation in an oncogene governing the cell signal pathway.* CML also demonstrates multistep carcinogenesis. The *BCR/ABL* event characterizes the chronic phase of CML, but something else must happen to push the disease into the blastic phase. A number of "second" events have been found in blast phase, including an additional chromosome 8, as in our case example. Frequent mutations in p53 or N-*ras* have also been found, acquired as the disease moves from chronic to blast phase.

Bone Marrow Transplantation

Chronic myeloid leukemia was for many years refractory to therapy. Hydroxyurea could decrease the white blood cell count, but did not appear to prolong the chronic phase or overall survival. Within the last 10 years, treatment with interferon has been found to be effective in producing complete remission in a substantial fraction of patients. In patients who respond, the blood and bone marrow become normal appearing, and the Philadelphia chromosome is no longer detectable by karyotype or Southern blot. However PCR, which can detect 1 cell in 10,000, frequently shows a low level of persistent leukemia in these patients. This very minimal residual disease does not necessarily lead to relapse. Whether interferon alone will produce long term cures is still under clinical study.

Bone marrow transplantation from an HLA-matched or partially matched donor is a more difficult therapy than interferon, but does offer a significant chance for cure. Molecular probes have allowed us to follow what happens following a bone marrow transplant. The interaction of the tumor and the immune system is particularly intriguing. Bone marrow transplantation following pretreatment with chemotherapy and total body irradiation reconstitutes both the hematopoietic and immune systems of the host patient with donor cells. After transplantation the following tissues in the host will have become reconstituted from donor cells: (1) the hematopoietic system including platelets, red blood cells, and granulocytes; (2) B and T lymphocytes, both in blood and lymph nodes; and (3) the monocyte-macrophage system including blood monocytes, tissue and alveolar macrophages, Kupffer cells of the liver, central nervous system glial cells, bone osteoclasts, and dendritic Langerhans cells of the skin.

At the moment of transplantation, the bone marrow and lymphoid tissues of the host are dying due to chemotherapy or irradiation given pre-transplantation. The patient becomes pancytopenic and severely immunocompromised. The production of new platelets, granulocytes, and red blood cells derived from the growing transplanted donor marrow occurs relatively quickly and approaches normal levels within 14 to 30 days posttransplant. During engraftment we have a mixing of the immune system of the host with that of the donor. Even in a good HLA match there will be immune reactions. The most important is **graft versus host disease (GVHD)**. The transplanted immune system of the donor recognizes the host as foreign tissue and attempts to "reject" the host. Immune reactions characterized by lymphocytic infiltration of the skin, liver, and gastrointestinal tract are common. Immunosuppressive therapy, sometimes long term, is necessary to control GVHD. Some attempts have been made to avoid GVHD by pretreating the donor marrow to eliminate T-cell function. However, these clinical trials soon led to the observation that when no GVHD occurs, relapse of the leukemia is more likely. We now appreciate that bone marrow transplantation in leukemia is more than just reseeding the hematopoietic system after high dose chemotherapy. Bone marrow transplantation is also immune therapy. Specifically, GVHD acts to kill leukemic cells that remain after chemotherapy (see Chapter 11). Using either PCR or FISH as sensitive methods to detect small numbers of residual *BCR/ABL* positive leukemic cells, we see that the leukemia persists for months after transplant. The disappearance of residual *BCR/ABL* positive cells appears to require GVHD.

A long unanswered question in cancer biology has been, is there any immune surveillance against tumor cells? These observations about GVHD being necessary to clear out residual CML suggest that at least in special circumstances, there is immune surveillance. Whether the body's immune system normally works to eliminate leukemic or other cancer cells remains unknown.

Similar Molecular Events in Three Types of Lymphoma

The molecular evolution of lymphomas reenforces the lessons learned in CML with some interesting variations. Lymphocytes are the only cells in the body that normally rearrange their genetic material.* However, the

---

*That is to say, as far as we know. The diversity provided by gene rearrangement is astronomical. I expect to see gene rearrangement discovered in other complex cell systems, such as the central nervous system.

rearrangement of immunoglobulin genes in maturing lymphocytes is in-efficient with lots of errors. Usually the errors are discarded by the mech-anism of cellular apoptosis. Occasionally an oncogene is involved in the error; this results in a tumor. First, I will describe normal immunoglobu-lin gene rearrangement in lymphocytes. Then, we will examine three types of lymphoma, each of which involves a tumor suppressor gene or an onco-gene erroneously joined to the immunoglobulin gene. The molecular events are only slightly different in each type of lymphoma, but the re-sulting clinical behavior is very different.

Immunoglobulin Gene Rearrangement in Lymphocyte Differentiation

As lymphocytes differentiate from a precursor cell, they rearrange their immunoglobulin genes to produce a specific antigen. Think of the 100 or so genes in the immunoglobulin gene families as a deck of cards. Each mature lymphocyte is one deal of about ten cards from this deck. From the repertoire of 100 or so immunoglobulin genes, millions upon millions of different antibodies can be produced. Each is a different deal of the cards, a unique gene rearrangement for each specific antibody. This is how the immune system is able to respond to so many different antigens using only a small number of genes.

Mature B lymphocytes produce an immunoglobulin that consists of two heavy chains and two light chains (of either kappa or lambda subtype). Figure 7.3 shows the steps in the rearrangement of the heavy chain por-tion of the B-cell immunoglobulin chain genes on chromosome 14. Genes

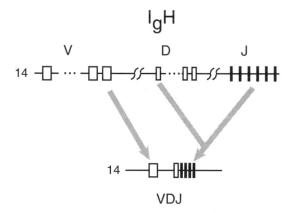

FIGURE 7.3. The heavy chain of immunoglobulin is formed by the fusion of exons from multiple subfamilies on chromosome 14.

must be joined from the V, D, and J families to produce a rearranged *VDJ* gene that codes for the heavy chain. The *VDJ* piece will then be joined to the C or constant region. The rearranged immunoglobulin heavy chain is frequently denoted as **IgH**. As a pre-B lymphocyte in the germinal center of a lymph node or the bone marrow differentiates, it first splices several of the six J segments to several of the greater than 20 D segments. The genetic material between the splice is discarded. Next a few of the greater than 50 V segments are joined to the DJ piece. Again the spliced out genetic material is discarded. The maturing lymphocyte can never reverse its destiny. It has permanently given up large parts of its immunoglobulin genes. It is now committed to producing only one specific antibody. The same gene rearranging happens for the kappa light chain genes on chromosome 2 and for the lambda light chain genes on chromosome 22.

By now you might be thinking, this seems a little complex. It is. A lymphocyte only succeeds in being its own genetic engineer about one time in three tries. Normally, lymphocytes that fail in their attempt at gene rearrangement undergo apoptosis. However you can see the potential for trouble. All these splices are just begging for an oncogene to slip in place of an immunoglobulin gene and cause trouble. In Chapter 5, I mentioned that occasionally one is driven to wonder why cancer does not occur every few minutes, given all the potential for errors. Fortunately repair systems are in place to remove these abnormal cells. Lymphoma happens, but considering the immense number of lymphocytes that develop normally, it is a rare event.

Burkitt's Lymphoma, t(8;14) t(2;8) t(8;22), and *myc*

Burkitt's lymphoma (small cell noncleaved lymphoma) is a high-grade malignancy that results from the insertion of the c-*myc* oncogene into the immunoglobulin gene during gene rearrangement. Three chromosomal translocations occur all producing the same result; the c-*myc* gene is spliced into the middle of an immunoglobulin gene. Figure 7.4 shows these three translocations: t(8;14), t(2;8), and t(8;22). These involve the heavy chain, kappa light chain, and lambda light chain genes respectively. In each case, we are left with a rearranged immunoglobulin chain gene that has the c-*myc* oncogene spliced in.

Think what happens. The lymphocyte's function is to produce immunoglobulin. When it tries, it instead produces c-*myc* mRNA. The c-*myc* gene is under the influence of the promoters and enhancers of immunoglobulin expression. c-*myc* is expressed inappropriately. Once expressed c-*myc* causes the cell to divide. This is the start of the malignant

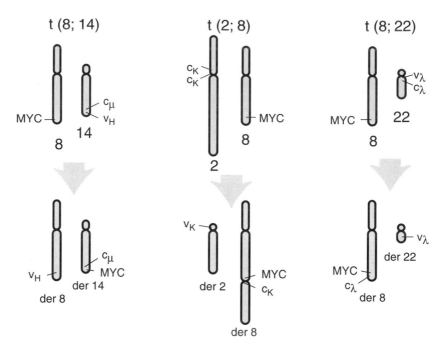

FIGURE 7.4. Three chromosomal translocations are seen in Burkitt's lymphoma. Each one results in the c-*myc* oncogene being fused with a portion of the immunoglobulin gene.

clone that results in Burkitt's lymphoma. Burkitt's lymphoma is a highgrade malignancy with rapid growth. This is not surprising. c-*myc* is a powerful stimulus to cell division.

The molecular evolution of Burkitt's lymphoma explains only part of the pathogenesis of this disease. It is important to recognize what we do not understand, even while we are enjoying the discovery of key molecular events. Burkitt's lymphoma occurs at a much higher frequency in immunosuppressed patients, especially T-lymphocyte suppression. Sir Denis Burkitt described the disease in areas of Africa with a high incidence of malaria. One could have asserted that mosquitoes "caused" lymphoma, although Burkitt, being a good epidemiologist, emphasized only the association. We now know that mosquitoes "cause" malaria. Malaria suppresses T-lymphocyte immune function. T lymphocytes help hold B- lymphocyte proliferation in check. When T-lymphocyte function fails, the incidence of Burkitt's lymphoma (and other malignancies) soars. This appreciation of the role of the immune system in holding B-cell clones in check was not understood until the era of AIDS. HIV infection, like malaria, suppresses T-lymphocyte function. Physicians knowledgeable about malaria correctly predicted that AIDS patients would also demonstrate a high incidence of Burkitt's lymphoma.

There is another important event in the pathogenesis of Burkitt's lymphoma, infection with Epstein-Barr virus (EBV). In Africa, virtually all infants have experienced EBV infection prior to age 1. EBV causes a polyclonal expansion of B lymphocytes. As immunity develops, this expansion is suppressed by T lymphocytes. When T immunity fails secondary to malaria, the EBV infected B lymphocytes again proliferate. A mistake in gene rearrangement produces a translocated c-*myc*. The breakpoint in the c-*myc* translocation is usually different in African patients (endemic Burkitt's) compared to non-African (sporadic Burkitt's). However, both demonstrate an overexpression of c-*myc*, resulting in a tumor.

What can be said to "cause" the tumor? Figure 7.5 demonstrates the multiple steps leading to endemic Burkitt's lymphoma. The first "causal" event is EBV infection, which occurs in infancy. The next "causal" event is the malarial mosquito that leads to suppression of T-lymphocyte function. This is followed by a chromosomal translocation that activates c-*myc*. So now what is your answer to what causes Burkitt's lymphoma?

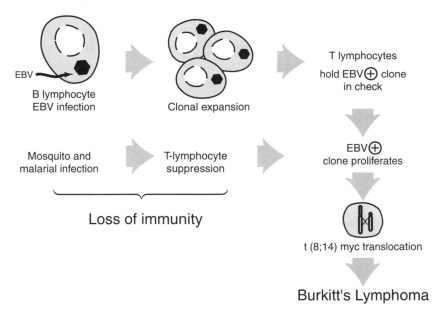

FIGURE 7.5. Multiple steps occur in development of endemic Burkitt's lymphoma, involving EBV infection, loss of T-cell immunity, and a chromosomal translocation.

In sporadic Burkitt's occurring in Western countries, the steps shown in Figure 7.5 are a bit different and the clinical disease is not the same. EBV infection does not occur in infancy (when the immune system is being schooled). Other factors in addition to EBV may provide the initial B-lymphocyte stimulation. Immunosuppression is due to AIDS rather than malaria. The c-*myc* translocation occurs in a later step in B-lymphocyte differentiation. The result is still a high-grade malignant lymphoma, but the classic presentation as a tumor of the jaw is rare.

In Chapter 5, our discussion of the role of the immune system in the multistep evolution of cancer was limited. We admired the complexity of the immune system and admitted that there is much we do not know. The development of Burkitt's lymphoma gives us additional information and clues. The activation of c-*myc* through chromosomal translocation starts a malignant clone. The status and past history of the immune system very much influences how that malignant clone will develop.

The diagnosis of Burkitt's lymphoma is usually straightforward based on examination of tissues or blood. The malignant cell, a small lymphoblast, has a characteristic morphology. Any gene probe that detects immunoglobulin or c-*myc* rearrangement will confirm the specific molecular lesion. A karyotype will demonstrate one of the specific translocations. In Chapter 11, we will discuss molecular anticancer therapies. Several ideas for therapy are suggested by what we now know about Burkitt's lymphoma. First, preventing and curing AIDS and malaria would very substantially reduce the incidence of this disease. Second, steps that down regulate immunoglobulin production by B lymphocytes might shut down the stimulation of the translocated c-*myc*. Finally, antisense oligonucleotides are a possible chemotherapy. The c-*myc* mRNA is fused to adjacent translated immune gene sequences in the tumor cells. An antisense oligonucleotide specific to the fused region might block c-*myc* expression uniquely in the tumor cells.

Mantle Cell Lymphoma, t(11;14), and *CYCLIN* D1

Mantle cell lymphoma is an intermediate grade, somewhat special form of lymphoma that is characterized by a specific chromosomal translocation. Once again the immunoglobulin heavy chain gene is involved. This time the "parasitic" gene that splices into the heavy chain gene is ***CYCLIN*** **D1** also called *PRAD* or *bcl*-1. The IgH/*CYCLIN* D1 fusion gene results in an overexpression of cyclin D1 protein. This protein stimulates cells to cross the G1/S boundary.

Like c-*myc*, *CYCLIN* D1 is a stimulus to cell proliferation, but rather more subtle or gentle. The substitution of *CYCLIN* D1 for c-*myc* in the fusion gene greatly changes the clinical nature of the resulting lymphoma. Mantle cell lymphoma follows a more indolent course with a relatively low proliferating fraction. Mantle cell lymphoma usually presents in the gastrointestinal tract. This form of lymphoma does not appear to be associated with EBV infection, nor is it more common in immunosuppressed patients.

The diagnosis of mantle cell lymphoma is sufficiently subtle, due to its close histologic resemblance to other forms of intermediate grade lymphoma, that I consider molecular confirmation necessary. A simple method is an immunohistochemical stain to detect the overexpression of *CYCLIN* D1. A karyotype of lymphoma cells demonstrating t(11;14) defines the diagnosis of mantle cell lymphoma.

Follicular Lymphoma, t(14;18), and *bcl-2*

A third chromosomal translocation involving the heavy chain of the immunoglobulin gene is t(14;18). This translocation is seen in most low-grade follicular lymphomas. The gene on chromosome 18 that is erroneously spliced into the IgH gene in this translocation is the *bcl-2* oncogene. Figure 7.6 is a gene map of the IgH/*bcl-2* fusion. There are at least two different breakpoints on chromosome 18, leading to different IgH/*bcl-2* fusion genes. The level of *bcl-2* mRNA is observed to vary significantly in cases of t(14;18) follicular lymphoma. Alternate splicing of the mRNA and influence of promoters or enhancers may be factors in *bcl-2* expression. There are a lot of details about the molecular biology

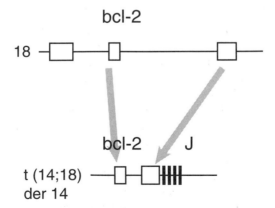

FIGURE 7.6. A gene map of the IgH/*bcl-2* fusion shows the result of a t(14;18) chromosomal translocation as seen in follicular lymphoma. The fusion gene is an error that closely simulates normal immunoglobulin gene rearrangement.

that are not certain. What we do know is that expression of *bcl*-2 blocks apoptosis! In Chapters 2 and 4, *bcl*-2 in apoptosis was stressed as one of the important genes in regulating the growth of tissues. This is especially true for lymphocytes in which apoptosis is a frequent means of removing cells.

Follicular lymphoma is a low-grade, indolent tumor. Molecular probes for *bcl*-2 rearrangement, usually using a PCR method or FISH, or a method of demonstrating *bcl*-2 overexpression, improve the accuracy of diagnosis. The tumor cells in follicular lymphoma have a very low proliferative fraction, nearly zero. However, they hang around nearly forever, having an even lower apoptotic fraction. Follicular lymphoma does not respond very well to chemotherapy based on drugs toxic to dividing or metabolically active cells. Antisense oligonucleotides are again a possible new therapy (see Chapter 11). Other means of influencing lymphocyte proliferation using cytokines also suggest new ideas for therapy. The fact that the abnormal lymphocyte in lymphoma is a member of a distinct clone raises the possibility of immunotherapy. A monoclonal antibody against the CD20 antigen (Rituximab, Idec Pharmaceuticals, San Diego) on B lymphocytes has recently been approved for lymphoma therapy. We may be able to engineer an even more specific antibody designed to be cytotoxic to just the tumor. This would require molecular engineering of an antibody specific for each patient. Biotechnology has reached the point where this is possible.

Summary

Leukemia and lymphoma demonstrate the molecular basis of cancer in an attractive but deceptively simple manner. An oncogene such as myc *is translocated into the immunoglobulin gene. The lymphocyte tries to make an immunoglobulin but instead produces* myc *protein. This forces cell division. A high-grade Burkitt's lymphoma is the result. We can even enjoy the illusion that we know why the chromosome translocation occurs in the first place. The lymphocyte must rearrange its immunoglobulin gene and, in so doing, it opens up all those "sticky" DNA splice acceptor sites.*

However, clinical knowledge of lymphoma suggests that the whole story is necessarily more complex. Burkitt's lymphoma is quite rare in non-EBV infected, nonimmunocompromised patients. Yet we all rearrange very large numbers of lymphocyte immunoglobulin genes every day in response to antigenic stimulation. As we learned in Chapter 5, cancer is a multistep process. Even in leukemia and lymphoma, where

*the signal molecular event is so straightforward, other factors modu-
late the development of disease. In the next chapters, we shall see this
multistep development of cancer become progressively more detailed.*

References

Groffen J, Stevenson JR, Heisterkamp N, et al. Philadelphia chromosomal breakpoints are clustered within a limited region, bcr, on chromosome 22. *Cell.*
1984;36:93–99.

Jandl JH, ed. *Blood.* 2nd ed. Boston: Little, Brown; 1996:903–923.

Kantarjian HM, O'Brien S, Anderlini P, Talpaz M. Treatment of chronic myel-
ogenous leukemia: current status and investigational options. *Blood.* 1996;87:
3069–3081.

Nowell PC, Hunderford DA. A minute chromosome in human chronic granulo-
cytic leukemia. *Science.* 1960;132:1497.

Sokol JE, Cox EB, Baccarani M, et al. and the Italian Cooperative CML Study
Group. Prognostic discrimination in "good-risk" chronic granulocyte leukemia.
Blood. 1984;63:789–799.

Voncken JW, Kaartinin V, Pattengale PK, et al. BCR/ABL P210 and P190 cause
distinct leukemia in transgenic mice. *Blood.* 1995;86:4603–4611.

Colon Cancer

Overview

Colon cancer has a well defined, multistep evolution defined both by histology and by molecular events. Colon cancer occurs both in an hereditary pattern secondary to germline mutations and, more commonly, in a sporadic pattern secondary to somatic mutations. The molecular lesions of colon cancer appear years before invasive cancer. The cells lining the colon are bathed in a lifelong effluent of bacteria and breakdown products of digestion. Our knowledge of carcinogenesis agrees with epidemiologic evidence that suggests a high-fiber, lower-fat diet would decrease the incidence of colon cancer. Inert fiber moves stool through the colon faster, decreasing exposure of the lining cells to carcinogens. Less fat and more antioxidants in our diets may further shift the rate of carcinogenesis. (Recall the steps in Figure 5.2.)

An important goal is to discover a molecular screening for colon cancer that is simple and effective. The detection of oncogene mutations in DNA shed from premalignant colon polyps in a stool sample promises to provide the PAP smear for colon cancer. Blood tests for inherited mutations in tumor suppressor genes define people at significant risk who will benefit from frequent colonoscopy. The molecular biology of colon cancer also suggests molecular therapies to treat metastatic disease. One approach is to attack cancer cells deficient in p53 gene function. Our understanding of colon cancer is more advanced than our understanding of most cancers. Hopefully what we are learning will be applicable to cancers of the pancreas, lung, prostate, and other tumors.

Hereditary Colon Cancer

About 15% of colon cancers have a hereditary component due to a germline mutation in a tumor suppressor or DNA repair gene.* The genes that are mutated in hereditary colon cancer overlap considerably with the mutations that are seen in the more common sporadic cases. Table 8.1 lists the genes involved in colon cancer, according to our current knowledge. We will discuss them in detail as this chapter develops.

In the hereditary **familial adenomatous polyposis coli (FAP)**, the *APC* tumor suppressor gene on chromosome 5 is mutated by deletion. The *APC* gene has a region within its main coding sequence in exon 15 in which most mutations are clustered. Mutations further towards either end of the *APC* gene produce a milder form of the syndrome. The disease is not manifest immediately because the patient also possesses a normal wild-type allele. With time, loss of heterozygosity (LOH, see Chapter 4) causes both copies of the *APC* gene to be mutated within increasing numbers of cells. The colonic mucosa develops hundreds to thousands of adenomas (polyps). This happens in the second decade of life, with the problem worsening as the patient ages. The polyps progress to cancer by the pathway to be discussed in the next section. Removal of the colon is necessary to prevent cancer.

Another well recognized predisposition to colon cancer is **hereditary non polyposis colon cancer (HNPCC)**. The germline mutations in this disorder occur in a group of genes called **mismatch repair genes**, examples of which are h*MSH2* and h*MLH1*. The mismatch repair genes may be considered as either DNA repair genes or a class of tumor suppressor genes. Again, LOH is necessary before any defect in DNA repair occurs. Tumor cells from patients with the HNPCC syndrome demonstrate **microsatellite instability**. A microsatellite is a repeat DNA sequence such as <u>CAGT</u>CAGTCAGTCAGT. Sometimes the repeat is just one base pair like AAAAAAAAAA. With loss of the mismatch repair genes, the length of these repeated sequences is not maintained. The microsatellites are scattered throughout the entire genome. When their length starts to vary, mutations occur in adjacent genes. Eventually an oncogene or a tumor suppressor gene is affected.

---

*This figure of 15% may change. As we find more genes involved in the evolution of cancer, we have new targets to examine for a hereditary component. Also, the incidence of hereditary versus sporadic tumors vary for different ethnic groups. Ashkenazi Jews have a higher hereditary incidence for both colon and breast cancer.

Table 8.1. Genes implicated in colon cancer.

Inherited
Hereditary non polyposis colon cancer (HNPCC)
Mismatch Repair Genes: h*MSH2* h*MLH*1
h*PMS*1/h*PMS*2
Familial adenomatous polyposis coli (FAP)
APC
Other hereditary forms
11307K (present in Ashkenazi Jews)

Somatic mutations
APC
K-*ras*
MCC
DCC
p53

These two syndromes, APC and HNPCC, account for only about one-third of colon cancers with an hereditary component. A recently discovered mutation in codon 1307 of the *APC* gene, designated mutation 11307K (Laken et al., 1997) does not produce the FAP syndrome, but does increase the risk for colon cancer. The mechanism of how this mutation leads to cancer is intriguing, and serves as an example of a more subtle hereditary predilection for cancer. The 11307K mutation changes a piece of DNA from AAATAAAA to AAAAAAAA, i.e., a T to A transversion. DNA does not like stretches of one base repeated many times. Enzymes that copy, translate, and repair DNA get confused by a stretch of As. The 11307K mutation is not so bad in itself, but it produces a hypermutable state that leads to further mutations. This unstable piece within the *APC* gene eventually leads to nonfunction of this tumor suppressor gene and colon cancer. The 11307K mutation occurs in 6% of Ashkenazi Jews, but very rarely in other ethnic groups.

The total percent of colon cancers that have an hereditary component is between 5% and 30%. Our rapidly increasing knowledge of the genes listed in Table 8.1, and the likelihood that others will be discovered makes this important number uncertain. Any system of screening for colon cancer must take into account the hereditary component. Patients at increased risk due to germline mutations require closer observation. For the FAP syndrome, resection of the colon is indicated. For other mutations where the risk is less than 100%, further observation is required. We do not yet have the experience to be specific. We will again encounter this uncertainty in the degree of risk of inherited mutations when we look at breast cancer in Chapter 10. Right now, a physician can send a blood sample to the laboratory to detect germline mutations responsible for FAP and HNPCC syndromes. Like the test for the breast cancer susceptibility genes *BRCA*1 and 2, we have a laboratory result before we have the clinical experience of what to do.

Molecular Evolution of Colon Cancer

Colon cancer starts as a polyp that enlarges and becomes more dysplastic. Carcinoma *in situ* within a polyp precedes early invasive cancer, which in turn precedes metastatic disease. A rough estimate is that polyp-to-cancer takes five years. The Dukes and TNM staging systems for colon cancer *begins* with early invasion. Molecular staging of colon cancer recognizes a number of stages occurring years before invasive cancer.

Colon cancer demonstrates more clearly than any other tumor the multiple molecular steps from normal, to neoplastic, and then to invasive cancer. In the preceding section we considered patients with germline mutations in tumor suppressor genes that lead to an inherited pattern of colon cancer. In the more common sporadic form of colon cancer, the process follows the same evolution. It just takes longer because the first step has not happened at birth. Figure 8.1 shows a pathway for the molecular evolution of colon cancer involving at least 5 mo-lecular stages. A diagram similar to this figure is standard in any article discussing the molecular events in colon cancer. The idea that colon cancer is a multistep evolu-

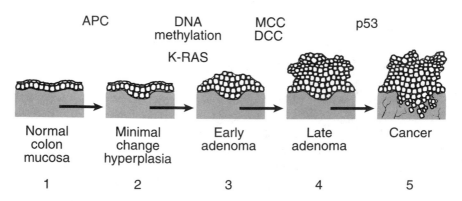

FIGURE 8.1. The molecular evolution of colon cancer is a series of mutations that parallels histologic changes.

tion should come as no surprise to readers of this book. This is the key concept that we have been developing. We will see in the following discussion that we must begin to incorporate this concept into our clinical thinking about cancer patients.

The molecular evolution of colon cancer diagrammed in Figure 8.1 begins with the deletion of part of the *APC* tumor suppressor gene on chromosome 5. The loss of the protective function of the tumor suppressor gene occurs only when both alleles are damaged through the mechanism of loss of heterozygosity. At this early stage, we may see no change from normal in examining the colon mucosa. Possibly a minimal amount of hyperplasia of the epithelial cells will be present.

The next stage is a change in the methylation pattern of DNA within the nuclei of the colon epithelium. Methyl groups can be attached to nucleotides, like pasted notes on a memo. The nucleotides of DNA are variably methylated based on the cell's past history. DNA that has been "read" tends to be more meth-ylated. Methylation events are a factor in regulating gene expression. Another event, also detected at this stage (#3 in Figure 8.1) is a point mutation in K-*ras*. By now the process is visible as an adenoma when viewed through an endoscope and biopsied. The patient is not likely to have any symptoms from this small adenoma. However an adenoma will likely progress if not removed.

The next stage (#4) is a larger villous adenoma that disrupts the colon architecture. This late stage villous adenoma may produce a small amount of chronic blood loss and symptoms consisting of a change in bowel habits. This stage is associated with LOH and function loss due to deletion of the *DCC* (deleted in colon cancer) gene on chromosome 18 or the *MCC* (missing in colon cancer) gene on chromosome 5.

Untreated, the late stage villous adenoma has a high probability of progressing to an invasive colon cancer (stage 5 in Figure 8.1). Invasive colon cancers almost always have a deletion mutation in the p53 tumor suppressor gene. Invasive colon cancer cells demonstrate a number of additional changes. They are capable of invading surrounding stroma, presumably due to a loss of cell surface receptors that serve as tissue anchors. The tumor cells elicit angiogenesis to supply blood to the growing tumor mass.

The molecular scenario depicted in Figure 8.1 is a common pathway in colon cancer. Other gene mutations can occur that will lead to the same result. There are not always five molecular stages. Table 8.1 lists more genes that have been found to be mutated in colon cancer, and this list will certainly grow. Other combinations of multiple molecular events offer different paths to the same biologic outcome. Colon cancer does not always progress through the stages of early and late adenomas as recognized by histology. However, the picture of the evolution of colon cancer that I have drawn in Figure 8.1 is a consensus of the findings of many researchers. This is how it happens much of the time.

Carcinogenesis and Colon Cancer

The molecular evolution of colon cancer as depicted in Figure 8.1 describes what happens but not why. Why does K-*ras* suffer specific point mutations, and why does the *APC* gene become partially deleted? There are no complete answers to the why of mutation in colon cancer, but our knowledge of the process of carcinogenesis gives some suggestions. The columnar epithelium lining the colon turns over rapidly with a relatively high mitotic rate. The cellular lining of the gastrointestinal tract must undergo renewal to compensate for functional wear and tear. These dividing cells are exposed to a mixture of bacterial and digestive breakdown products. In the colon, feces remain in contact with the epithelium for hours to a few days. Many of the organic breakdown products in feces are mutagenic in vitro, and presumably carcinogenic in vivo. Thus the setting in the colon is one of chronic exposure of dividing cells to carcinogens. This satisfies most of the criteria for effective carcinogenesis.

What can we do to decrease tumor development in the colon? Sir Denis Burkitt, whose epidemiologic studies showed the role of malaria in lymphoma, also noted a large variance in the incidence of colon cancer relative to the amount of indigestible fiber in the diet. In India and other Eastern countries, colon cancer is much less common than in Western countries. One hypothesis is that a high fiber diet leads to a rapid transit of feces through the colon. Chronic exposure to the carcinogens in feces is decreased by rapid passage of stool through the colon. The diet of these Eastern cultures, besides including more fiber, is low in animal fats and high in vegetables and fruits. The breakdown of fats produces carcinogens. Vegetables and fruits contain antioxidants and free radical scavengers that detoxify carcinogens. Recall Figure 5.2, a diagram of the steps of carcinogenesis. Improved diet can decrease the amount of carcinogens and increase the rate of their detoxification. We can measure this. Biopsies of the colonic mucosa of persons on diet A (high fiber and antioxidants, low fat) should demonstrate fewer DNA adducts than those in people with a typical Western diet. Epidemiologic studies commonly use disease incidence as an endpoint in assessing risk factors. The detection of DNA adducts as a premutation event is an endpoint in carcinogenesis of the colon that precedes clinical disease by probably a half a decade or more.

Screening and Early Detection

The clinical management of colon cancer seeks to prevent invasive disease by screening for polyps and removing them via colonoscopy. This is considerable progress from pre-endoscopy days of twenty years ago. We seek to treat colon cancer before it becomes cancer. Regrettably, colonscopy screening is invasive and expensive. Many patients present with advanced disease.

Our knowledge of the histologic and the molecular evolution of colon cancer suggests improvements in screening. There are two screening strategies in current widespread practice: (1) testing of stools for occult blood, and (2) colonoscopy. The detection of occult blood in stools is inexpensive, but inefficient at detecting early colon neoplasms. In fact, the fecal occult blood test (FOBT) is not so inexpensive because it is inefficient, leading to expensive work-ups in false positive cases. True positives are all too often late stage disease. Polyps are not likely to bleed unless they are large or already invasive cancer. On the other hand, screening colonoscopy is efficient but expensive. A new approach is to detect mutated oncogenes or tumor suppressor genes in stool samples.

The K-*ras* oncogene demonstrates point mutations in a majority of villous adenomas. This mutation occurs at an early step as demonstrated in Figure 8.1. This is usually before a polyp is large enough to cause symptoms. A molecular screening test using PCR to detect K-*ras* mutations in stool should detect colon polyps at an earlier stage than the current testing of stools for occult blood. DNA is fortunately a very robust molecule. Sloughed and autolyzed cells from a polyp provide fragments of DNA that can be detected with high sensitivity by PCR even in the "dirty" background of digested fecal material. Early clinical trials suggest that this method is feasible. The detection of deletions within tumor suppressor genes in stool samples is more difficult. DNA in stool is fragmented. DNA fragments are a suitable substrate for PCR detection of simple point mutations. The genomic sequencing necessary to find variable and complex deletions in tumor suppressor genes would be difficult in stool specimens. Extensive clinical trials will be necessary to learn the sensitivity and specificity of any molecular based screening test. The good news is this. *All of our examples of the multistep molecular evolution of cancer teach us that gene mutations precede clinically recognizable disease.* Colon cancer is a testing ground for new molecular screening methods. Polyps detected early can be removed by endoscopy and invasive cancer avoided. By the new criteria of outcomes, this is a very desirable result.

Molecular Staging

We have long recognized the multiple stages in the progression of cancer. Clinical staging has been a significant goal for many years. To compare treatments, patients must be of equal clinical stage. Molecular biology has discovered that cancer begins as a noninvasive clonal proliferation of cells with specific molecular lesions. In Figure 8.1, we considered five molecular steps, the first four of which proceed what we call cancer. We will need to incorporate this knowledge into our clinical staging of cancer. Table 8.2 is an example of a molecular staging system for colon cancer, alongside the TNM and Duke's classical staging.

The molecular stages are defined according to which oncogenes or tumor suppressor genes are mutated. A person who inherits a deletion in the *APC* gene, as for example in the FAP syndrome, starts life at the first molecular stage. A person who has a positive screening test for K-*ras* in a stool sample is at the next molecular stage. If a colon polyp is found at colonoscopy, and the polyp has a deletion in the *DCC* gene then the stage is again moved up. A villous adenoma with carcinoma *in situ* that also demonstrates loss of function of p53 is where the molecular classification begins to overlap with the first stage of the TNM or Duke's classification. Table 8.2 is a proposal for the molecular staging of colon cancer. Any such system will have to be validated with clinical experience, as was done for the TNM classification. The advantages of adding a molecular stage to precancerous lesions follow the same arguments used decades ago for the classical TNM system. Molecular staging, if validated

Table 8.2. Classical and molecular staging of colon cancer.

Histological stage	Molecular stage	TNM stage	Dukes stage
Normal	—	—	—
Minimal change	*APC*	—	—
Early adenoma	*ras*	—	—
Late or villous adenoma	*DCC, MCC*	—	—
Carcinoma *in situ*	p53	0	—
Carcinoma, invading mucosa	—	I	A
muscularis propria	—	II	B
Carcinoma, metastatic to regional	—	III	C
lymph nodes distant sites	—	IV	C

in clinical trials, will allow us to compare the effectiveness of new schemes for screening and treatment.

Molecular Therapies

The molecular biology of colon cancer has identified specific mutations that are the cause of the malignant behavior of the cells. A far more lofty goal than merely detecting the lesions is to fix them! Molecular therapies for cancer are the most exciting outcome of DNA technology. Molecular therapy, which we will consider more broadly in Chapter 11, is in its infancy. Some examples of new ideas for the treatment of colon cancer will, however, show the potential of this approach.

Adenovirus Killing of p53 Deficient Tumor Cells

Most colon cancers (and 50% of all cancers) have a mutation in the p53 tumor suppressor gene. Recall from Chapters 2 and 4 that the normal function of p53 system is to detect abnormal or damaged DNA. The p53 gene then holds these damaged cells up at the G1/S phase boundary in the cell division cycle until the damage is repaired (Figure 4.3). If the repair is not made, the cell undergoes suicide through apoptosis. Adenovirus, the infectious agent that causes many minor upper respiratory infections (colds), has genetic machinery that allows it to subvert p53 function in the human cells. When adenovirus invades a cell, it is detected as abnormal DNA. However, the virus has a gene that allows it to override the p53 checkpoint. The cell is forced to manufacture many viral copies.

These traits of the adenovirus have been adapted to make it an antitumor agent. A genetically engineered adenovirus that does not have the capability to overcome the human p53 gene has been created as an anticancer agent. This strain (O15 Onyx Pharmaceuticals Richmond, Ca) can only propagate in p53 deficient cells. Cancer cells are p53 deficient! Thus cancer cells are the targets for infection by this strain of adenovirus, where normal cells are spared. When O15 infects cancer cells, it overwhelms the cancer cell with viral copies. The cancer cell then lyses releasing virus to infect other cancer cells.

The strategy to use genetically engineered adenovirus to infect p53 deficient cancer cells is very clever. Clinical trials are underway or planned for colon, head and neck, ovary, and pancreas cancers. We will need experience with this new kind of therapy, but the prospect is exciting. A few limitations can be imagined. The body mounts a very effective defense against adenovirus through the immune system. Adenoviruses are overcome in a few days via neutralizing antibodies produced by B lymphocytes. Will the immune system stop the beneficial infection of a genetically altered adenovirus? Can we take steps to limit the body's defenses against adenovirus to make the infection persist? The O15 strain of adenovirus may not be the magic bullet that kills all p53 deficient cancer cells. However, the idea to use a biological vector to kill selectively based on the damaged genome present in cancer cells is a powerful example of biotechnology and molecular based therapy.

p53 Antibodies

Loss of p53 function is so common in many types of cancer that much therapy has been targeted at this defect. Another approach, currently being widely explored, is antibodies to p53 protein. Cancer cells with deletions in the p53 gene overexpress a nonfunctional form of the protein. Figure 8.2 is a photograph of a colon polyp stained with an antibody to p53. The neoplastic cells show strong staining, while normal colon epithelium is negative. The infusion of antibodies to p53 protein should attack these neoplastic cells. Various tags can be applied to p53 antibodies to make them toxic to tumor cells. Radioactive, chemical, or immuno-

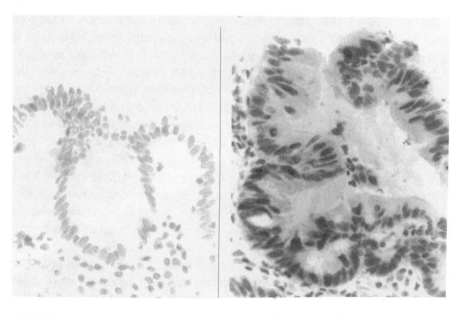

FIGURE 8.2. A colon polyp stained with an antibody to p53 shows abnormal accumulation within neoplastic cells (right panel), but negative staining in the normal mucosa (left panel).

logic tags are being used. Clinical trials of anti-p53 antibody for metastatic colon cancer are underway (see Chapter 11).

Summary

Colon cancer demonstrates the multistep evolution of cancer in terms of histology and molecular lesions. Neoplastic clones of cells progress over years through four or five well defined stages before they become colon cancer. We can see the results of carcinogens at work in molecular lesions of colon mucosa. This makes possible new methods to survey the effects of diet and other chemoprevention strategies. The detection of mutated oncogenes is a tool for molecular screening to detect precancerous colon polyps. The ultimate goal, however, is to fix molecular damage. A genetically engineered adenovirus that attacks p53 deficient cancer cells is one approach. Antibodies to p53, which is overexpressed in tumors, is another. The key concept of this chapter is embodied in Figure 8.1. Cancer develops in a series of molecular steps. For colon cancer, we have come a long way in determining what those steps are.

References

Bischoff JR, Kirn DH, Williams A, Heise C, Horn S, Muna M, Ng L, Hye JA, Sampson- Johannes A, Fattaey A, McCormick F. An adenovirus mutant that replicates selectively in p53-deficient human tumor cells. *Science.* 1996; 274:373–376.

Giardiello FM, Brensinger JD, Peterson GM, et al. The use and interpretation of commercial APC gene testing for familial adenomatous polyposis. *New Engl J Med.* 1997;336:823–827.

Laken SJ, Petersen GM, Gruber SB, et al. Familial colorectal cancer in Ashkenazim due to a hypermutable tract in APC. *Nature Genetics.* 1997; 17:79–83.

Tomlinson I, Ilyas M, Novelli M. Molecular genetics of colon cancer. *Cancer and Metastasis Rev.* 1997;16:67–79.

Squamous Cell Carcinoma
of the Uterine Cervix

Overview

"Squamous cell carcinoma of the uterine cervix is caused by a virus and may be cured by a vaccine." To be more precise, let me rephrase that to say: Human papilloma virus (HPV) is a common initiating factor in the cascade of molecular events that leads to squamous cell carcinoma of the cervix. A vaccine that impedes HPV should decrease the incidence of cervical cancer. This chapter discusses viral carcinogenesis. We will find that host factors affecting HPV infection modulate the likelihood of cancer. Again, we will prove the maxim that cancer develops in multiple steps over a period of years.

Epidemiologists look at cancer as a series of factors that affect the incidence of disease. Radiation is linked to an increase in leukemia and low-fiber diet, to a decrease in colon cancer. In cervical cancer, the majority of disease is linked to HPV infection. The PAP smear has given us a window to observe the progression of cellular dysplasia to cancer. We know that HPV-infected cells will show dysplastic changes over time. This dysplasia is reversible and most patients revert to normal. In the small percent of patients who progress to high-grade dysplasia and invasive cancer, additional unknown factors must be at work. A vaccine that impedes HPV should reverse the initiating step in the progression to cancer. An HPV vaccine must be DNA based as opposed to a protein antigen in order to induce T-lymphocyte mediated cellular immunity. The T-cell response is necessary to fight the virus in its intracellular location. The future will likely see molecular detection of HPV supplementing the PAP smear as a screening method. A bioengineered DNA vaccine will help prevent or reverse dysplasia.

Cytologic Progression of Cervical Cancer

Squamous cell carcinoma of the uterine cervix takes years, even decades, to progress from the earliest histologic abnormality of low-grade dysplasia to invasive cancer. Sound familiar? This is very similar to the development of colon cancer as we saw it in the last chapter. Again, we are looking at cancer as a multistep evolution over years. There are many gaps in our knowledge about cervical cancer; but what is known is very intriguing. The PAP smear has been our principal tool for observing the cervix, and the results of cytology have established the dogma surrounding this disease. Within the endocervical canal, the epithelium of the cervix makes an abrupt transition from squamous to columnar. The PAP smear samples cells shed from this transition zone as the epithelium renews itself. Inflammation and hormonal influences alter this sharply defined transition zone.

About 15% of women demonstrate some abnormality in maturation of the squamous epithelium as seen on PAP smear. The terminology to describe the progressive stages of cytologic abnormality is dictated by the Bethesda system in an attempt to avoid numerous overlapping terms. Minimal disruption of normal cytology is called *ASCUS* (*atypical squamous cells of uncertain significance*). Figure 9.1 is a schematic of the stages in the Bethesda system for describing progressive dysplasia. In the next section, evidence is presented to demonstrate that most cases detected as ASCUS represent HPV infection of the squamous epithelium. The women who demonstrate ASCUS/HPV generally go onto LGSIL (low-grade squamous intraepithelial lesion). The mean time for progres-

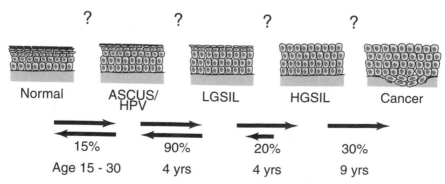

FIGURE 9.1. A diagram shows the progression of cervical dysplasia through the stages recognized by the Bethesda system for PAP smears. The time spans and probabilities for passing between stages is indicated at each step.

sion from ASCUS to LGSIL is about 4 years. Patients with LGSIL usually revert to normal without treatment. Only about 20% of LGSIL cases
continue on to the next stage, HGSIL (high-grade squamous intraepithelial lesion). This progression also takes about 4 years. HGSIL is also called
severe squamous dysplasia or *carcinoma in situ*. HGSIL is probably not
reversible. Some studies suggest that a small percentage of HGSIL patients untreated may spontaneously revert to lower grade lesions. However
HGSIL is not usually left untreated. At this stage, an excisional cone
biopsy of the dysplastic epithelium results in cure. In most HGSIL patients, if no treatment is given, progression to microinvasive and then to
deeply invasive squamous cell carcinoma occurs with a time lag of roughly
9 more years. Figure 9.1 summarizes this progression. The diagrams at
the top of the figure are stylized sketches of the squamous epithelium at
each stage in the progression towards cancer. Dysplasia is the histologic
term that includes the changes of LGSIL and HGSIL. In dysplasia, the
squamous cells from the basal layer fail to mature as they age and migrate towards the superficial layer. They also demonstrate nuclear atypia
characteristic of HPV infection.

Time Course of Cervical Carcinogenesis

Many factors are thought to induce dysplasia. Infection with the human
papilloma virus (HPV) is undoubtedly by far the most common. Dysplasia
develops in a high percent of individuals with HPV detected on the cervix.
Some patients with dysplasia will return to normal; others will progress
to high-grade lesions and cancer. In Figure 9.1, very approximate esti-
mates are given for the percent of cases that progress to the next stage as
well as the mean time span for that progression. Figure 9.2 demonstrates
additional evidence that helps us understand the time course of HPV progressing to cancer. The incidence of HPV infection, cervical dysplasia,
and invasive cancer of the cervix are plotted as a function of age. The
Y-axis on this graph is not to scale for the three populations. Each successive step has a lower incidence. About 15% of women will at some
time in their life have detectable HPV on a cervical swab, with the incidence peaking between 15 and 30 years of age. The molecular methods
for detecting HPV (to be discussed in more detail later) have varying sensitivity, and the true incidence of HPV infection is uncertain. Like all sexually transmitted diseases, the incidence of HPV has increased over the
last several decades. Dysplasia, usually detected as LGSIL or HGSIL on
a PAP smear occurs in as many as 90% of HPV infected individuals, with
a peak incidence between 25 and 45 years. Invasive squamous cell car-

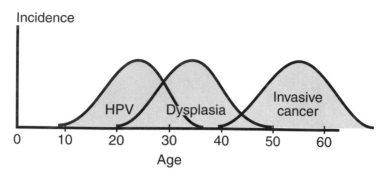

FIGURE 9.2. The incidence of HPV, dysplasia, and invasive cancer as a function of age shows the slow development of cervical cancer.

cinoma of the cervix should be a rare disease. Its incidence is a reflection of the effectiveness of screening programs. The incidence is low in women who have had frequent PAP smears. Severe dysplasia in these patients is treated before it can become cancer. Cancer, when it does develop, has a peak incidence between 45 and 65 years of age. The time course for cervical carcinogenesis as reflected in Figures 9.2 and 9.1 applies to most cases of HPV induced dysplasia followed by squamous cell cancer. The dysplastic epithelium is derived from a single mutated cell and the squamous dysplasia is clonal and thus a true neoplasm (as defined in Chapter 5). However, multiple lesions, each derived from alternate clones, may be present simultaneously. The steps demonstrated in Figure 9.1 are analogous to the multistep evolution of colon cancer that was shown in Figure 8.1. However we do not have a good understanding of the molecular lesions that accompany each stage in Figure 9.1. At each transition, I have indicated a "?" For the multistep development of colon cancer in Figure 8.1, specific gene lesions are listed. A study of the molecular biology of HPV shows a less complete understanding of the specific genetic lesions leading to cervical cancer.

Molecular Biology of Human Papilloma Virus (HPV) and Cervical Cancer

The human papilloma virus (HPV) contains circular, double-stranded DNA, 7900 bp in length contained within a capsid. There is no outer envelope, which makes the virus somewhat labile to the environment. There are at least 70 strains of HPV with different disease causing potential.

HPV infects epithelial cells by direct contact and is thus predominantly a sexually transmitted disease. HPV infection in the genital region causes symptomatic warts (condyloma) or more commonly results in an asymptomatic infection. Urogenital warts are usually flat, sometimes not easily recognizable, especially on the penis. HPV infection outside the urogenital area results in the common papillomatous skin wart. The warts due to HPV infection usually spontaneously resolve. Clinical treatment if necessary is simple mechanical or chemical removal of the tissue, although immunotherapy with interferon is also used.

The viral genome depicted in Figure 9.3 begins with a control region that contains regulatory genes. These regulatory genes help the virus use some of the infected cell's machinery for replication of the virus. For example, one of these genes is a promoter gene sensitive to the cell's RNA polymerase. Thus the machinery within the cell for transcribing and translating DNA to RNA to protein can be used by the virus for replication. This is a common mechanism in viruses that replicate within a host cell. The virus can have a much smaller genome, since it "borrows" gene functions from the cell. Downstream (clockwise in Figure 9.3) from this control region is a long open reading frame (ORF) that encodes genes con-

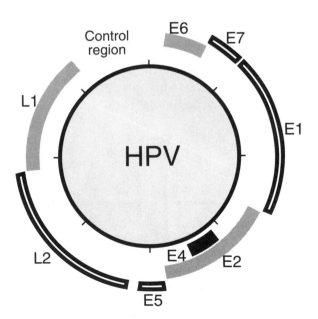

FIGURE 9.3. A genome map of HPV reveals early and late transcribed genes, and a region for controlling gene function. The HPV genome is in the form of a circle, 8000 bp in circumference.

trolling viral growth as well as the viral structural proteins. These genes are divided into early (E) and late (L). The L1 and L2 genes encode proteins for the viral capsid.

Two of the HPV genes, E6 and E7, are of special interest to us. These genes have transforming or oncogenic potential for human cells. The E6 and E7 proteins can inactivate the proteins from the human tumor suppressor genes p53 and *RB* as we discussed in Chapter 4 and especially Figure 4.3. When p53 protein is inhibited by interference from the E6 protein, the infected squamous epithelial cell can enter the S phase of the cell division cycle without being checked. With p53 inhibited by HPV, the cell's entrance into S is deregulated, greatly increasing the possibility that errors in DNA synthesis will occur with resulting mutations. The E7 protein has a similar interaction with the *RB*1 tumor suppressor gene function. Again, the viral protein inhibits tumor suppressor gene function and leads to the potential for more mutations as the unchecked squamous epithelial cells proliferate. Figure 9.4 is a schematic summarizing the inhibition of p53 and *RB*1 by HPV E6 and E7 proteins. This is a case of inhibition of inhibitors leading to promiscuous proliferation!

Life Cycle of HPV Infection

So far the story of HPV induced carcinogenesis of the cervix is coming together too well. I do not believe that I have emphasized enough that other variables, especially host factors, greatly influence the outcome of HPV infection. This section on the life cycle of HPV infection will more clearly demonstrate the gaps in our knowledge. Figure 9.5 is a schematic of the possible events occurring in the basal squamous epithelium of the

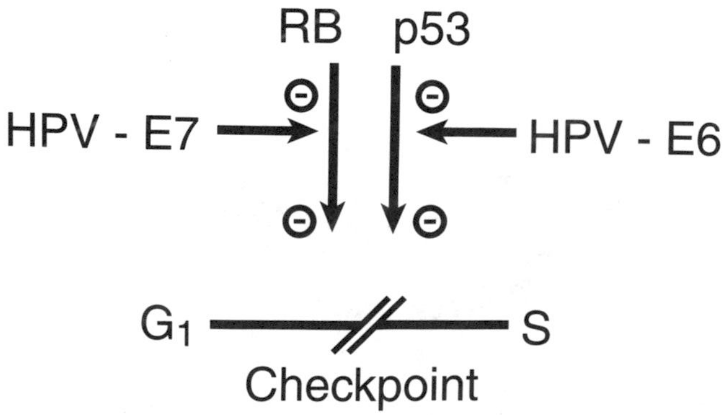

FIGURE 9.4. The E6 and E7 HPV proteins inhibit function of p53 and *RB* tumor suppressor genes in the cells infected with the virus.

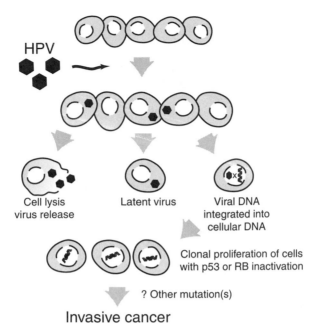

HPV

Cell lysis
virus release

Latent virus

Viral DNA
integrated into
cellular DNA

Clonal proliferation of cells
with p53 or RB inactivation

? Other mutation(s)

Invasive cancer

FIGURE 9.5. The HPV viral life cycle includes three phases: immediate cell lysis with release of virus; a latent viral infection; and integration of HPV DNA into the cellular DNA. The later step is necessary for viral carcinogenesis.

uterine cervix following HPV infection. There are multiple paths, only one of which leads to cancer. We do not understand fully the host and viral factors that determine which path HPV infection will take. Starting at the top of Figure 9.5, I have indicated that exposure of the squamous epithelium to HPV results in infection of a certain percent of basal cells. We can detect this infection by *in situ* hybridization with molecular probes for HPV. Figure 9.6 is a photomicrograph of the *in situ* detection of HPV in a cervical biopsy. We know a significant percent of women will have HPV infection during their life. The HPV infected basal epithelial cells can follow several different courses. In an active or production infection, propagation of virus inside the cell leads to cell lysis and release of free viral particles (left path in Figure 9.5). The virus may also enter a latent phase, not replicating or doing anything, just hanging around in the cell's cytoplasm (center path). Eventually this cell will likely mature becoming an anucleate shed squamous cell. This would clear the virus from the epithelium. The latent infection can also activate at some future time. The right hand path in Figure 9.5 demonstrates the most important outcome, integration of the viral DNA into the cell's genome. This step is impor-

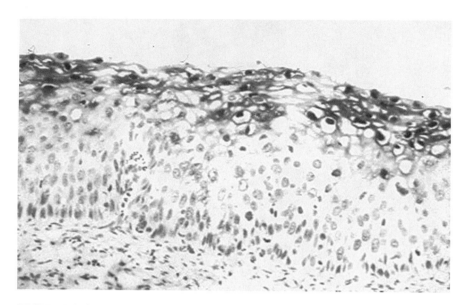

FIGURE 9.6. A photomicrograph of an *in situ* molecular probe for HPV strain 18 demonstrates intracellular virus in this cervical biopsy. The dark staining nuclei in the vacuolated cells of the upper level of the epidermis are positive.

tant for viral induced carcinogenesis. The suppression of tumor suppressor genes by the virus and the possibility for induction of mutations due to viral insertion into the cellular DNA are carcinogenic events.

We do not know what factors favor integration of viral DNA into the cell's genome. Possibly one of the more important factors is HPV type. Table 9.1 lists a number of strains of HPV and their association with risk for cervical cancer. The high risk strains show stronger binding of E6 and E7 proteins to the tumor suppressor genes. Viral load at the initial infection and host resistance will also influence the outcome.

The start of a clonal neoplasm follows the integration of HPV DNA into the cell's genome. Squamous cell dysplasia is a clonal neoplastic process. We can tell this from the signature of each single virus entering

Table 9.1. HPV types and cervical carcinoma risk.

HPV Type	Risk	Viral protein/ tumor suppressor gene interaction	
6,11	Low	E6 does not bind p53	E7 weak binding to Rb
31,33,35,51,52	Intermediate		
16,18,45,56	High	E6 binds p53	E7 strong binding to Rb

the cellular DNA at a slightly different location. Multiple dysplastic clones may coexist indicating that initiation of neoplasia following viral integration is reasonably common. These clones over a time span of very roughly 9 years lead to invasive squamous cell carcinoma. Other mutations are undoubtedly responsible for the progression of the multistep carcinogenesis. We have not as yet discovered them. Host factors are also an issue. Immune suppression, such as AIDS, substantially accelerates the development of cervical dysplasia.

Molecular Detection of HPV

The molecular detection of HPV is a straightforward problem. The genome of HPV (Figure 9.3) contains sequences that are unique to this virus. More specific portions of the genome differentiate the various strains. It is possible to construct molecular probes that will cover many strains or be targeted at only one strain such as the high risk HPV 18. After designing the probe, the next choice is sensitivity of detection. A PCR detection system with amplification of virus can signal the presence of only a few virus particles in a cervical swab specimen. Less sensitive are *in situ* hybridization methods that detect heavily infected cells in a PAP smear or a cervical biopsy. Figure 9.6 is a photomicrograph of HPV *in situ* hybridization on a cervical biopsy. The cells labeled with black granules contain virus. The peroxidase labeled HPV DNA probe has bound to target sequences on the virus. We visualize the probe by carrying out a color reaction that makes the peroxidase label stain darkly. We can "see" the virus within squamous cells in the biopsy in Figure 9.6.

The sensitivity of HPV detection is an issue. PCR methods detect an HPV positive rate of 10% to 15% in US women. Less sensitive *in situ* hybridization show less than half as many affected. Is there a threshold for number of virus particles, below which HPV is not likely to induce the changes shown in Figures 9.1 and 9.2? Certainly in addition to the number of virus particles, host factors such as immune status, hormonal status, and other coexisting diseases will influence whether HPV infection occurs. *In situ* hybridization demonstrates that HPV has entered the cell. This combined with observing the cytology changes of ASCUS, LGSIL, or HGSIL confirm HPV induced cervical disease. A labeled HPV probe has been FDA approved (Digene, Beltsville MD). Clinical trials will take some time to determine how to use HPV molecular detection results. The combination of a molecular method for HPV detection and the PAP smear should allow for more accurate classification of which women are at risk for developing cervical carcinoma.

Anti-HPV Vaccine as Treatment and
Prevention for Cervical Cancer

The immunity necessary to provide protection for some viruses is not easily obtained. Most traditional vaccines are derived from a piece of the viral coat. Killed virus is injected as a foreign antigen to invoke an antibody response. Protein as an antigen invokes humoral immunity. Immunoglobulin in the serum and on the surface of B lymphocytes is the antibody. Humoral immunity fights free virus in the blood stream. However, HPV spends most of its life cycle inside a squamous epithelial cell. This hides it from humoral antibody attack. A new class of vaccines based on DNA are being studied for intracellular viruses with a latent phase of infection. **DNA vaccines** have the potential of invoking cellular immunity. DNA vaccines require a vector to carry the DNA into the cell. These vaccines may use live virus vectors, or at least an "active" vector to carry the DNA across the cell membrane. Once inside the cell, the engineered pieces of DNA in the vaccine code for viral proteins. The production of these proteins intracellularly is what leads to T-lymphocyte mediated cellular immunity.

DNA vaccines offer the potential to treat and provide immunity against a number of microbial and viral illnesses for which current vaccines are unavailable. These include HPV, HIV, and Helicobacter pylori. The vaccines being studied include live and dead viruses, and engineered pieces of DNA administered orally, topically, and injected.

We commonly think of vaccines as useful only as a preventive measure, to be given before the infection occurs. HPV is a chronic infection. A DNA vaccine that induces T-lymphocyte immunity has plenty of time to alter the course of the disease. Several anti-HPV vaccines are in various phases of development and clinical trials. Most are given only to women with HPV infection. Prophylaxis in women not infected is something that will likely be left for the future. The questions to be answered by a clinical trial are, does the vaccine reverse the infection (as indicated by an appropriate molecular test)? Does the vaccine reverse or prevent the development of LGSIL or HGSIL? The answers to these questions are not yet known.

Summary

Squamous cell carcinoma of the cervix demonstrates a stepwise progression of molecular lesions similar to colon cancer. The initiating event in most instances is HPV infection. The virus interferes with p53 and RB1 tumor suppressor gene function in the infected squamous cells.

This allows other mutations to go unrepaired and the damaged cell to avoid destruction by apoptosis. Multiple clones of squamous dysplasia are the result. These clones will progress to carcinoma over a time span of years if they are not removed. Molecular probes that detect HPV strains associated with a high risk of dysplasia can augment the PAP smear in screening strategies. A DNA-based vaccine against HPV inducing cellular immunity might be the best treatment and prevention for this cancer. This cancer, caused by a virus, will likely be the first cancer cured by a vaccine.

References

Barbosa MS. The oncogenic role of human papillomavirus proteins. *Critical Reviews in Oncogenesis.* 1996;7:1–18.

Demay R. *The Art and Science of Cytopathology. Exfoliative Cytology.* Chicago: ASCP Press, 1996:97–108

Prasad CJ. Pathobiology of human papillomavirus. *Clin Lab Med.* 1995;15:685–704.

Shroyer KR, Thompson LC, Enomoto T, et al. Telomerase expression in normal epithelium, reactive atypia, squamous dysplasia, and squamous cell carcinoma of the uterine cervix. *Am J Clin Pathol.* 1998;109:153–162.

Breast Cancer

Overview

Breast cancer is our fourth and final clinical example of the principles of molecular oncology. In the previous chapters on leukemia/lymphoma, colon cancer, and squamous cell carcinoma of the cervix, we saw several common threads. Tumors develop as the result of a germline or somatic mutation in a tumor suppressor gene or oncogene. Invasive cancer is the endpoint of a multiple-step evolution that can be tracked as a series of progressive histologic and molecular lesions. Breast cancer demonstrates these common principles, but the details are less clearly understood. What percent of cases is due to inherited risk (germline mutation) versus sporadic breast cancers (somatic mutation)? At the moment, we can estimate the inherited risk as 5% of breast cancers. But this estimate is likely to change as we discover more of the genes involved. What are the steps in evolution? Under the microscope we recognize the progression of hyperplasia, atypical hyperplasia, in situ carcinoma, and invasive cancer. The molecular evolution of breast cancer is less clearly understood. The linear sequence of molecular events that we saw in Figures 8.1 and 9.1 for colon and cervical cancer may not exist in as simple a form for breast cancer.

Breast cancer makes us face the complexity of a disease modulated by host factors. Age, hormonal status, immune status, and other unknown factors appear to affect the incidence and aggressiveness of breast tumors. The current staging of breast cancer, more than any other tumor, takes this into account. A number of tumor and host parameters are collected in an attempt to predict the aggressiveness of each individual case. The success of these additional parameters in improving prognosis or adjusting therapy is much debated. Progress in the treatment of breast cancer has been primarily in early detection. Breast cancer (like colon and cervical cancer) is cured by surgical excision in the early clinical stages. Metastatic breast cancer is usually fatal. This leads us to a tactical plan to develop better screening. Genetic testing for breast cancer susceptibility by sequencing BRCA*1 and* BRCA*2 genes is a test case for genetic screening in general. How do we use this new genetic information? The treatment of metastatic breast cancer requires new molecular therapies to supplement radiation and chemotherapy if we are to improve survival rates.*

Molecular Pathology

The female breast undergoes a great deal of growth, differentiation, and remodeling beginning at puberty and continuing until menopause. The tubules and ducts of the breast are lined by columnar epithelium. This tissue proliferates and regresses under the hormonal influence of the menstrual cycle and local growth factors. Unlike the endometrial lining, the breast epithelium is not sloughed off and replaced at each menstrual cycle. The breast epithelium has a lot of history behind it as the years progress. The development of breast cancer is related to history. Age at menarche, age at birth of first child, number of children, use of hormonal birth control, age at menopause, and hormone replacement therapy have all been related to the incidence of breast cancer.

We have discovered a number of genes that are mutated in breast cancers. I have given a partial listing in Table 10.1. This list includes oncogenes like ***her-2/neu***. This gene is mutated by the mechanism of gene amplification in about 25% of breast cancers. The *her-2/neu* gene is a membrane growth factor receptor. Amplification of the gene results in overexpression of receptors on the tumor cell surface. This was one of our models of molecular mutations leading to cancer that we discussed in Chapter 3, specifically in Figure 3.3b. Other oncogenes such as c-*myc* and *INT*2 are also found amplified in a significant percentage of breast cancers. Activation of a proto-oncogene to its oncogene form by the mechanism of gene amplification seems to be more common in breast cancer than other tumors that we have studied. In Chapter 3, gene amplification was mentioned as a type of mutation, but only briefly. We do not know what causes gene amplification. The development of microsatellite repeats is perhaps a similar phenomenon. The formation of these short repeating sequences is a sign of genomic instability, usually due to a failure of repair secondary to loss of tumor suppressor gene function. It will be important for us to find out what tumor suppressor genes besides *BRCA*1 and 2 are mutated as an early step in breast cancer.

Table 10.1. Genes involved in breast cancer.

Oncogenes	
Cyclin D1	Limits cell cycle progression in G1 phase; affected by hormonal status; gene is amplified and protein overexpression in some tumors
her-2/neu	Transmembrane receptor, overexpressed in some tumors; may indicate drug resistance
INT2	Mutated from proto-oncogene to oncogene in some tumors
c-myc	"
c-ras	"

Tumor suppressor genes	
p53	Loss of function in many tumors, increased proliferation and mutation
RB	"
?maspin	A possible tumor suppressor gene that functions through preventing tumor cell invasion of the extracellular matrix

Other genes	
Cathepsin D	Interacts with basement membrane, overexpression in some tumors related to invasion
E-cadherin	Cell adhesion molecule, loss of expression in some tumors possibly related to invasion or metastasis
MDR-1	Multiple drug resistance gene, amplified in some tumors, pumps drug out of cell

One study (Deng et al., 1996) demonstrates a method for discovering early tumor suppressor gene mutation in breast cancer. These investigators studied loss of heterozygosity (LOH) in normal appearing breast glands adjacent to invasive carcinomas and carcinoma *in situ*. They performed microdissection to remove histologically normal appearing tissue at the edge of a tumor. Using PCR they probed for mutations at several genetic loci including p53, *RB*1, as well as loci at chromosome map positions 3p24 and 11p15.5. They found six of ten cases demonstrating LOH at 3p24 establishing this site as a presumptive location for a tumor suppressor gene. The fact that these investigators found genetic mutations in normal appearing tissue is gratifying. Our theory of carcinogenesis suggests that early molecular lesions are the first steps.

The genes listed in Table 10.1 are probably only some of the genetic lesions that will eventually be discovered as the steps in breast cancer. If our list of potential genes is large, then the multistep genetic evolution of breast cancer will be complex and varied. We perhaps should not expect that a relatively simple set of successive steps will describe the molecular pathology of breast cancer. There may be many alternative pathways. As we shall see in the next section, breast cancer is characterized by a wide spectrum of clinical behavior. Our hypothesized multiple pathways may explain why cancers that appear histologically similar, behave differently.

Staging and Multiple Prognostic Factors

Breast cancer varies greatly in its aggressiveness. This has engendered a complex staging system to improve prognosis and choice of therapies. When invasive breast cancer is detected, staging involves determining: the maximum size of the tumor, the histologic grade of the tumor (architecture of glands, nuclear atypia, and number of mitoses), the presence and number of axillary lymph node metastases, and the presence of distant metastases. This basic staging data set establishes the traditional TNM stage. When patients are grouped according to TNM stage, the variable behavior of breast cancer is reduced but is still quite pronounced. This has led to attempts to find other factors that might further improve the prognostic value of staging. Table 10.2 lists a number of the factors that have been considered, beginning with our classical TNM stage, and then listing tumor cell and host factors that may be prognostic. Current clinical practice in staging breast cancer is evolving as we attempt to assimilate all these factors.

The problem in utilizing multiple new prognostic factors in breast cancer is that a factor that is a strong predictor in one clinical situation may be of very limited value in another. It would make good sense that measuring the number of *her*-2/neu growth factor receptors would predict the "biological" aggressiveness of an individual tumor. In clinical trials, overexpression of *her*-2/*neu* is associated with a poor prognosis. But this is true only in patients with the histology of ductal carcinoma who are axillary lymph node positive. In other clinical situations *her*-2/neu status is not clearly predictive. Another example is overexpression of cathepsin-D. This protease is overexpressed in some tumors, but usually only in patients who have positive axillary lymph nodes. In fact, the correlation between axillary lymph node status and cathepsin-D is so strong that cathepsin D is not an independent factor. It probably only reflects the presence and number of axillary lymph node metastases. The measurement of tumor cell proliferation, determined as the S phase fraction (SPF) is a third example (recall Figure 6.1). This parameter is an independent

Table 10.2. Prognostic factors in breast cancer.

Classical pathologic stage (TNM)
    Size
    Histologic type and grade
    Axillary lymph node involvement
    Distant metastases

Cellular characteristics
    Extensive *in situ* component (EIC)
    Proliferative rate
    DNA ploidy
    Estrogen and progesterone receptors
    Oncogene and tumor suppressor genes
    Other gene mutations

Host factors
    Patient age
    Hormonal/menopausal status
    Immune status

---

prognostic factor in patients who have no axillary lymph node metastases. S phase fraction performs even better as a prognostic factor in patients who also have small tumors.

You and I are, of course, most interested in the molecular factors that may affect the clinical behavior of breast cancer. We have already admitted that we do not know the molecular pathogenesis of breast cancer. Maybe we can gain some knowledge through a sort of molecular epidemiology. We will measure everything we can and see how it correlates with clinical outcome. When we do measure as many things as possible, the interaction between the various parameters becomes complex. To use the data, we must have a staging system that matches this complexity. The use of a **neural network** to handle the large number of interacting parameters has been tested with some success. Figure 10.1 is a very simplistic diagram of a neural net for breast cancer staging. This figure illustrates only seven tumor and host factors, each having six connections to the other members. A more realistic neural net would model many more parameters. Data based on measurements performed in a large number of patients is then fed into a computer. The computer simulates neural network interactions with each factor, enhancing or inhibiting the others. The computer considers all possible interactions until the data best fits the clinical outcome. As we gather more or new data the neural net adapts. This is more complexity than we are used to handling in clinical situations.

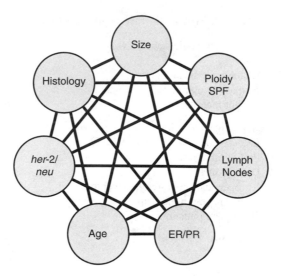

FIGURE 10.1. A neural net analysis of seven tumor and host factors models the complex interaction of parameters observed in breast cancer.

We have to become more sophisticated and accept complexity! For the moment, we can appreciate that aneuploid tumors with a high SPF are likely to be biologically aggressive. Such tumors will likely have loss of p53 or *RB* tumor suppressor gene function. Otherwise they would not have been able to accumulate all of the mutations that lead to aneuploidy! If the tumor expresses estrogen receptors, this means it still retains some normal response to hormones, and this can be used as therapy. We are making some progress with the biology of breast cancer.

Breast Cancer "Field Effect"—A Special Problem

Lobular carcinoma *in situ* (LCIS) is a specific histologic change in the breast epithelium that demonstrates the special problem of field effect. The breast is constructed of ducts and lobules surrounded by connective tissue and fat. Cancer more frequently develops within the ductal elements. Invasive ductal cancer represents the majority of breast tumors. A patient with a small ductal carcinoma can be treated with lumpectomy to remove the tumor, axillary dissection to assess the presence of lymph node metastases, and radiation and chemotherapy as indicated based upon staging data. The patient may also be treated with mastectomy if the tumor is larger or if the patient prefers this to adjuvant radiation therapy. For LCIS this approach does not work. A patient with LCIS or invasive lobular cancer has a high probability of recurrent cancer developing in either breast. LCIS is a marker of a "field effect." This poorly understood condition implies that throughout both breasts premalignant changes have occurred that will result in cancer within the next decade. The molecular basis of this change within the breast epithelium has not yet been discovered. Does it mean that very many epithelial cells have each suffered mutations? Could it mean that the breast epithelium in patients with LCIS is already a clonal neoplasm, *in both breasts*? Could it mean that whatever mutation is affecting the breasts is capable of transfecting nearby tissue? Squamous cell carcinoma of the cervix demonstrates a field effect. Recall from Chapter 9 that dysplasia is a clonal process, but that multiple simultaneous clones are common. This is driven by HPV infection. Is a similar undiscovered process occurring in lobular carcinoma *in situ* of the breast?

Breast cancer also demonstrates dramatically the problem of tumor heterogeneity. Most cancers show some difference in the degree of differ-

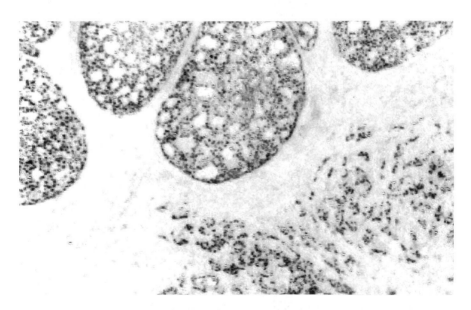

FIGURE 10.2. Immunohistochemical staining for estrogen receptors demonstrates the heterogeneity of intraductal (upper left) and invasive (lower right) components of breast carcinoma.

entiation of the tumor cells. We assign tumor grade based on the area with the worst histology. In breast cancer we frequently see a very wide range of differentiation. Often large areas around the invasive tumor have changes of carcinoma *in situ*. Everything we wish to measure in breast cancer is affected by tumor heterogeneity. Figure 10.2 is a photomicrograph of a breast cancer stained with an antibody to the estrogen receptor (ER). This is how we determine if a tumor is ER positive, i.e., do the tumor cells still have estrogen receptors? Note that the normal breast epithelium on the edge is strongly positive, portions of the tumor with *in situ* carcinoma are weakly positive, and the invasive tumor component is negative. In such situations we report the tumor as ER negative, since we judge the result on the worst histology. This heterogeneity makes measurement of parameters like ER or *her-2/neu* more difficult. Again the molecular pathology associated with tumor heterogeneity is uncertain. We may have multiple neoplastic clones with different molecular stages.

Breast Cancer Susceptibility Genes

Our first gene map in Chapter 1 was of *BRCA1*. We have come a long way since then. Gene maps are familiar to us now, and the information they impart is clearer. Let's revisit the breast cancer susceptibility genes, *BRCA1* and 2, in light of our increased knowledge and desire for clinical relevance. Figures 1.3 and 1.4 show *BRCA1* as a complex gene, with 23 exons. We know that over 200 different inherited mutations in *BRCA1* result in a high probability of breast cancer in the women who have a mutation.* Our scientific understanding of *BRCA1* is incomplete but emerging. *BRCA1* is a tumor suppressor gene in that the absence of its normal function results in a high incidence of tumors. The *BRCA1* protein is found expressed in fetal tissues, where its function is poorly understood. Most mutations like del185AG, which was discussed in Chapter 1, result in a frame shift in the transcription of the genome into mRNA. The protein translated from this incorrect transcript usually truncates far short of the 1863 amino acid length of the normal *BRCA1* protein. We would expect this. Frame shift mutations introduce random stop codons into the mes-

---

*The incidence for breast cancer in *BRCA1* positive women was estimated at 85% when I began writing this book. Within less than 12 months, more studies involving more mutations in a much larger number of women have changed this important number to 50% to 60%. Remember that we have very little clinical experience with molecular medicine, and our data is exciting but unrefined.

sage, which terminate the translation of the protein. This is illustrated in Figure 1.5.

The frequency of the 200 plus known mutations in *BRCA*1 is fairly evenly distributed with no one or small group of mutations accounting for a high percentage of cancers. The incidence of del185AG is 0.9% in Eastern European Jews, but this mutation is extremely rare outside this group. The uneven distribution of *BRCA*1 mutations among different ethnic groups is typical of most genetic traits. The large number of possible mutations and the variable incidence associated with ethnic background makes the problem of genetic screening for *BRCA*1 very complex.

The detection of one specific mutation in *BRCA*1 is relatively simple. The classic but now outmoded Southern blot procedure can easily detect del185AG. Methods employing PCR with hybridization probes are faster. Using multiple primers, several mutations can be screened for in a single run. For a few specific mutations these methods will work as a clinical laboratory test. However, to screen women for all the possible mutations, it is necessary to sequence the *BRCA*1 gene or to assay the protein. New technologies, such as DNA on a chip (as discussed in Chapter 6), might make direct sequencing sufficiently inexpensive to permit widespread screening. An alternate approach is to detect abnormal truncated *BRCA*1 proteins produced by mutated genes.

Several companies offer *BRCA*1 mutation testing. They advertise their products to physicians. Clinical trials employing these new technologies are far from complete; clinical experience with the test results is virtually absent. There is no consensus on what should be done with a negative or positive test result. For a negative result, there is concern that a woman will feel that her chances of breast cancer are slight and forego recommended screening. For a positive result, the advice varies from radical to conservative: bilateral mastectomies and oophorectomies at an early age versus more frequent physical exams and mammography.

Telling a woman with a *BRCA*1 mutation that she has a high probability of developing breast cancer is a very dramatic outcome of a clinical laboratory test. The effect on a person's behavior, child-bearing plans, employment, and insurance are all unknown. The direct medical cost effectiveness of *BRCA*1 testing is uncertain. A complete screen of the *BRCA*1 genome is approximately the cost of a lifetime supply of mammograms. Which expense will reduce the morbidity and mortality of breast cancer more? All of these issues—from the direct scientific question of whether gene mutations can be accurately detected in a clinical laboratory test, to all of the secondary questions of what medical actions should follow a negative or positive result—remain incompletely answered.

Summary

Breast cancer unfortunately demonstrates how much we do not yet know about the molecular biology of cancer. I present breast cancer as an antidote to any smugness that may have resulted from the much clearer examples of the molecular lesions in colon and cervical cancer. Many genes are implicated in breast cancer, suggesting that breast cancer may be more heterogeneous than we currently appreciate, with multiple pathways leading to malignancy. Our current knowledge suggests that we need a more sophisticated staging system, possibly using a neural network to analyze the many factors. Genetic susceptibility to breast cancer due to inherited defects in BRCA1 and 2 tumor suppressor genes accounts for only a small fraction of cases. Nevertheless, genetic screening for breast cancer may become a test case for the use of gene technology in our current medical system.

References

Deng G, Lu Y, Zlotnikov G, Thor AD, Smith HS. Loss of heterozygosity in normal tissue adjacent to breast carcinomas. *Science.* 1996;274:2057–2059.

Kodish E, Wiesner GL, Mehlman M, et al. Genetic testing for cancer risk. How to reconcile the conflicts. *JAMA.* 1998;279:179–181.

Miki Y, Swensen J, Shattuck-Eidens D, et al. A strong candidate for the breast and ovarian cancer susceptibility gene *BRCA1. Science.* 1994;266:66–71.

Olopade OI. Genetics in clinical cancer care—the future is now. *N Engl J Med.* 1996; 335:1445–1456.

Shattuck-Eidens D, Oliphant A, McClure M, et al. *BRCA1* sequence analysis in women at high risk for susceptibility mutations. *JAMA.* 1997;278:1242–1250.

Molecular Anticancer Therapies

Overview

Cancer results from a series of gene mutations that disrupt normal controls on cell growth. It is worth repeating this definition now, near the end of the book, in order to focus our discussion of molecular anticancer therapies. The most important result of the discoveries of molecular biology applied to cancer is knowledge. Knowledge provides a rational basis for therapy. We want new therapies aimed at the molecular lesions we have discovered. The most direct approach is to fix the mutations in DNA through genetic engineering. If we cannot do that, we can try to block abnormal gene function by interfering with transcription or translation. Alternatively, we can intervene at a later step with antibodies to abnormal oncoproteins.

Antisense oligonucleotides are a new class of drug that block specific gene expression. We can make that block permanent by transfecting cells with the antisense sequence. We can also transfect cancer cells with engineered viruses that infect only cells with mutations in the p53 gene. Alternatively, the virus may carry an altered gene that induces apoptosis or makes the cell more susceptible to chemotherapy. Treatment with antibodies to p53 and RB1 oncoprotein is another approach. Blocking cell surface receptors like her-2/neu is yet another.

Biotechnology makes possible the production of specifically designed proteins. We can manufacture cytokines, hormones, and other factors that modify the biologic behavior of tumor and host. An example is antitumor angiogenesis factor. Genetic engineering allows for altering the immune system. Lymphocytes can be taught outside the body to induce a cytotoxic response to tumor-associated antigens. They can then be reinfused to carry out immune destruction of their target. In this final chapter, we consider examples of molecular anticancer therapy. This field is just developing. We want to see what is possible and get a sense of how far we can go. The exam-

ples chosen show the variety and the inventiveness of new molecular therapies. Clinical results with these new therapies are nearly nonexistent. My purpose in this final chapter is to prepare us for what is coming.

Molecular Targets in Cancer

In Chapters 3 and 4 we learned that mutations in oncogenes and tumor suppressor genes are the cause of neoplastic cell growth. In Chapter 5, we viewed cancer as a multistep process, where neoplastic clones became invasive tumors by further mutations and gaining the ability to overcome host factors. This gives us a lot of new targets for anticancer therapy. Figure 11.1 is a schematic of some of the molecular therapies that we might try.

We wish to block the function of overactive oncogenes and restore the function of damaged tumor suppressor genes. Antisense oligonucleotides

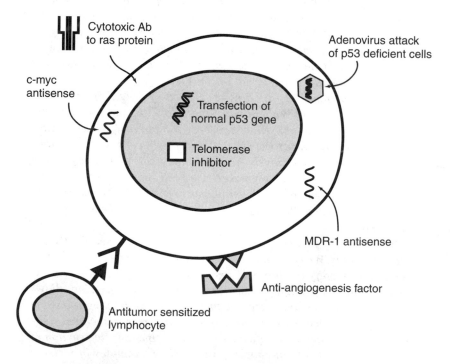

FIGURE 11.1. Molecular targets for anticancer therapy aim to correct, block, or destroy abnormal function.

(as we will discuss in the next section) give us a tool for inhibiting gene function. Transfecting cancer cells with normal tumor suppressor genes might restore them. We are talking about genetic engineering here! The cancer cell is damaged. We are going to set about fixing it. In Figure 11.1, I have indicated antisense to c-*myc*, antibody to *ras*, and transfection with normal p53 as examples of fixing the cell.

What we cannot fix, we wish to destroy. Cancer cells divide without aging. The telomeres at the ends of chromosomes do not shorten with each successive division (see Chapter 2). The enzyme telomerase that replicates these special DNA sequences is not suppressed in "older" cancer cells. Drugs that inhibit telomerase can take advantage of this difference. Many cancer cells are deficient in p53 function. In Chapter 8 we discussed a genetically engineered adenovirus that propagates only in p53 deficient cells. These are two more approaches diagrammed in Figure 11.1.

Table 11.1. Classes of molecular anticancer therapy.

Antibodies	
Anti-angiogenesis	Blocks tumor angiogenesis factors
Anti-CD20	Targets and destroys epitope on lymphoma cells
Anti-HER2	Blocks cell surface receptor
Anti-MDR	Blocks g170 glycoprotein and lowers drug resistance
Anti-p53	Attacks cells with overexpression of p53

Enzyme inhibitors	
Tyrosine kinase	Cell surface receptors
CDK	Cell cycle
Farnesyl transferase	Blocks *ras* protein binding

Antisense oligonucleotides	
bcl-2	Restores apoptosis
p53	Restores checkpoint
ras	Inhibits *ras* translation

Viruses	
p53	Restores wild-type tumor suppressor gene sequence
O15	Replicates in p53 deficient cells, causing tumor cell lysis

Vaccines	
anti-HPV	Induces cell mediated immunity to HPV

Cancer cells "know" that they are damaged. As we will discuss shortly, a gene system called multi-drug resistance (**MDR**) is stimulated in neo-plastic cells. The MDR function pumps out toxic molecules that build up in the cell's cytoplasm. Late stage cancers and cancer cells that have been exposed to chemotherapy have gene amplification of MDR. With this ad-ditional mutation, the cancer cell can pump out drug molecules faster than normal cells. This is the cause of acquired resistance to chemotherapy.

Our last steps in fighting the cancer cell lie in modifying host response. If we can block tumor angiogenesis, small tumors will starve themselves as they outgrow their blood supply. This has been an elusive, but still worthwhile, goal. Immune destruction of tumors does not often occur nat-urally. We are learning how to modify cells of the immune system out-side the body and then reinfuse them to kill tumors. Table 11.1 lists classes of molecular anticancer therapy with a few examples.

With all of these targets, how can we miss? Each area has significant technical problems. If we shut down all c-*myc* function with antisense, normal proliferating cells will also be severely restricted. Restoring tu-mor suppressor gene function by viral transfection seems like a great prospect. How can you have too much tumor suppression? Remember that we have just discovered tumor suppressor genes. We have no expe-rience with too much function. I can imagine holding up normal cells for too long at the G1/S checkpoint, until everything undergoes apoptosis! For every new therapy there are possibilities and problems. What is ex-citing is that we have so many new things to try. Let us now look at some areas in detail.

Antisense Oligonucleotides

A new class of drugs called antisense oligonucleotides can modulate the regulation of gene expression. When a gene is active, the first step in its expression is transcription of DNA to messenger RNA (mRNA). After transcription, the mRNA is exported from the cell nucleus into the cyto-plasm. There, the mRNA is bound to a ribosome and translated into a growing amino acid chain. The amino acid chain at the end of translation falls off the ribosome and folds into the protein that is the product of the transcribed gene. These steps are diagrammed in Figure 11.2.

Antisense oligonucleotides are a means for interfering with this process. A short piece of DNA, typically 15 to 30 bases long, is synthesized. This oligonucleotide is made as a complementary or genetic mirror image to a portion of the much longer mRNA molecule. This is called an antisense

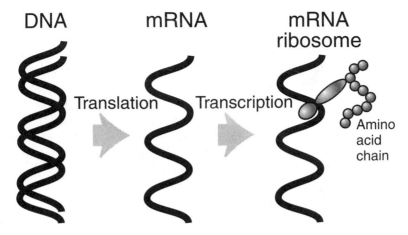

FIGURE 11.2. Gene expression begins with DNA translated into mRNA that is in turn translated into protein.

copy since it is complementary to the mRNA that contains the genetic message in the correct "sense" orientation. The antisense oligonucleotide binds to its complimentary target portion of the mRNA molecule and produces a short double-stranded sequence along this otherwise linear single-stranded molecule. Figure 11.3 shows an antisense oligonucleotide bound to mRNA. I have illustrated just 3 base pairs out of the 15 to 30 base pairings that hold the two strands together.

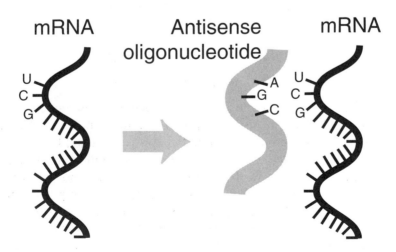

FIGURE 11.3. Antisense oligonucleotides bind to mRNA and block translation into proteins interfering with gene expression.

The double-stranded piece, resulting from the antisense oligonucleotide binding to mRNA, prevents translation into protein. Double-stranded RNA is recognized by the cell as abnormal and is destroyed by an enzyme called ribonuclease H. Alternatively, if the oligonucleotide targets a region near the 5' cap on mRNA, then binding to a ribosome is inhibited. The result of the antisense binding to mRNA is the functional destruction of that message. If the antisense is present in excess in the cytoplasm, no message can be successfully processed by the cell. Thus, despite the fact that a specific gene is turned on and actively being transcribed into mRNA, the message will not get through. In theory, antisense oligonucleotides are a very specific mechanism for interfering with the expression of only a single gene.

The blocking of gene expression by antisense oligonucleotides can be made permanent, rather than dependent on repeatedly dosing the cell with more drug. This is accomplished by transfection of an antisense sequence into a cell. Transfection with antisense sequences are a means of genetic engineering that may lead to the development of transgenic plants and animals with a resistance to pathogens.

Some important technical problems surround the use of antisense oligonucleotides as anticancer therapy. Oligonucleotides are intrinsically unstable, being rapidly degraded by enzymes within the cell and in the serum. Synthesis of new forms of antisense oligonucleotides with a modified chemical backbone offer increased stability and may overcome this normal degradation. In addition, antisense oligonucleotides are relatively large molecules with a molecular weight in the 5- to 15-kd range. This limits their ability to penetrate into the cell cytoplasm.

Immune Mediated Therapy

Antibodies to Oncoproteins

The p53 tumor suppressor gene and the *ras* oncogene are targets for antibody therapy because of their common abnormal expression in cancer cells. Recall that p53 protein is normally expressed only at low levels in cells in which this tumor suppressor gene is functioning. In neoplastic cells, mutations in p53 lead to abnormal protein that is not quickly degraded and thus overexpressed. Figure 8.2 shows a colon polyp stained with an antibody to p53. The adjacent normal colon mucosa is negative; the polyp is positive. The *ras* oncoproteins are also not normally expressed in tissues. Therefore, antibodies that elicit some sort of cytotoxic immune reaction to p53 or *ras* might selectively kill tumor cells. Since p53 and *ras* are not foreign proteins, the body does not normally make antibodies to them. They would be called tumor associated antigens (recall Chapter 5) since they are normal proteins, but abnormally expressed on cancer cells. We can attempt to immunize the patient to make antibodies to p53 and *ras*. An alternate approach is to produce antibodies outside the body and infuse them. Both approaches are being used in a number of clinical trials for metastatic breast, colon, and other cancers.

Graft versus Leukemia Therapy

An example that combines genetic engineering and immune mediated therapy is controlled graft versus leukemia therapy. Allogeneic bone marrow transplantation has demonstrated that an engrafted immune system provides a potent antileukemia reaction (see Chapter 7). Unfortunately this effect is directly linked to graft versus host disease, in which the graft reacts against the entire host as well as the leukemia. An experimental therapy to get the benefit without the side effect is the infusion of allogeneic, genetically engineered lymphocytes. A leukemia patient is matched to a donor who is compatible at major HLA histocompatible sites. The donor provides lymphocytes. These lymphocytes are genetically engineered in vitro by transfection with a thymidine kinase gene from the Herpes Simplex Virus (**HSV-tk**). The retroviral vector infects the lymphocytes and carries the gene into the lymphocyte genome. The altered donor lymphocytes are infused into the patient to establish a graft versus leukemia reaction. When it becomes necessary to halt the side effect of graft versus host, the antiviral drug gancyclovir is administered. The genetically altered lymphocytes containing HSV-tk are killed by gancyclovir. The immune match between donor and patient, the number of infused lymphocytes, and the dose of gancyclovir modulates the degree of the graft versus leukemia reaction. Thus, the reaction is controlled.

Genetically altered allogeneic lymphocytes are under development by Chiron (Emeryville, Ca). Chiron, in modern molecular biology jargon, has a **kit** for the HSV-tk retroviral vector. Kits are a common module in biotechnology, including the materials and, most importantly, the methods for carrying out a process. A complex piece of genetic engineering is accomplished by stringing together a series of kits. The HSV-tk retroviral transfection is a standard approach to genetically altering cells to make them susceptible to gancyclovir. This means the altered cells can be killed when necessary. An HSV-tk kit is to a genetic engineer as an amplifier module is to an electrical engineer. I cannot write about genetic engineering without thinking about some of the ethical and scientific dilemmas that are raised by this tool. Since we are talking about vaccines for treatment or prevention of cancer, let us take a moment to consider a side issue.

Infectious Vaccines—An Aside

Imagine the following scenario. Sometime in late 1999, a genetically engineered DNA vaccine for HIV is available. A United States-led international consortium of pharmaceutical companies announces that they can produce the vaccine for $20 a dose. They will distribute sterile single-dose injection units at cost on a priority basis, beginning with service to the countries that participated in the research and investment leading to the vaccine. The consortium anticipates production of 50 million doses the first year. The leader of a developing nation with a population of 120 million people, 20% of whom are infected with HIV, announces that this is unacceptable. This leader has recently come to power in a riotous revolution, in part a reaction to that country's health crisis. The health minister of this country, a highly respected physician, amplifies his president's comments by announcing that his country will soon begin release of an infectious *version of this vaccine. Working in a WHO laboratory that was taken over during the recent revolution, he and his colleagues have inserted engineered DNA that induces T-lymphocyte immunity to HIV into an influenza virus. The infectious virus carrying the DNA vaccine will soon be introduced into refugee camps located at this nation's borders. These refugees, 14 days after spread of the virus, will be released from the camps and allowed to return home. This, the health minister announces, is the only affordable and practical means of introducing the vaccine into the 120 million people of his nation. He also offers the modified influenza virus infectious vaccine to the health departments of other Third World countries.*

The scientific problems with the scenario outlined above are great, especially the risk of mutation in the infectious virus rendering it virulent instead of protective. Beyond the scientific problems loom far greater social and ethical issues. As the technical capabilities of molecular biology increase and become widespread, so do both the benefits and risks of its products. An infectious vaccine is a microbe designed to spread from person to person to induce immunity to a specific antigen. This is very close in technical specifications to an infectious agent designed to spread disease—an act of biological terrorism!

Many, if not most, people acquire immunity to viruses through subclinical or mild infections. In this sense, many people are immunized by an infectious "vaccine." Before the development of the vaccine for varicella, some parents intentionally exposed young children to the virus (chicken pox parties) so that they would have the illness at an age when it is usually mild. Some live vaccines in current use are infectious to un-intended hosts in the immediate family. The oral polio vaccine (OPV) oc-casionally spreads to parents of vaccinated children, causing the disease in an unprotected adult. The OPV is essentially the only source of the dis-ease, polio, in the Western world.

A novel vaccine derived from recombinant DNA that is not infectious, but is easily spread, is the hepatitis B banana. A protein from the coat of the hepatitis B virus has been inserted into the banana plant, creating a transgenic banana that expresses the virus coat protein in the edible fruit. Eating bananas from this plant provides immunization against the hepati-tis B. This novel vaccine was developed as a less expensive delivery sys-tem than the current series of three intramuscular injections. Widespread use of the hepatitis banana has not yet occurred. Will it be prescribed for individuals, *or released to protect* populations *at risk?*

The delivery of vaccines to large numbers of people is a complex and expensive task. The use of an infectious vaccine theoretically allows for inexpensive widespread delivery of the antigen. Plants and animals are treated with a wide array of vaccines where the target is the field or flock, not an individual. Salmon swim through chambers that topically apply vaccine for furunculosis. Poultry are vaccinated with aerosol sprays. Some secondary, infectious passage of a live virus vaccine occurs in agri-cultural usage. The appeal of an infectious vaccine is inexpensive, rapid, and wide dispersal of the antigen. An epidemic can be stopped before it spreads. The dangers are equally great; virulent mutations, uncontrolled spread, and unanticipated side effects.

Genetic Engineering

Any step that alters the genome of an organism can be considered genetic engineering. We have already considered many examples, such as the transfection of a thymidine kinase gene into a donor lymphocyte in order to make it sensitive to the gancyclovir. This is gene therapy. We have be-gun to use gene therapy in making the hematopoietic cells of a cancer pa-tient more resistant to the toxic effects of antimetabolite chemotherapy. This is done by extracting the bone marrow and transfecting it with an amplified *MDR*.

Genetic engineering crosses an invisible line and assumes a new mean-ing when we permanently alter the germline of an organism to create a "new" plant or animal. The day we alter the human genome in a germ cell, we will have changed our genetic destiny! The ability of humans to read and then finally to write our own genomes will change the way we see ourselves. The impact of such a change is beyond estimation. The day on which we do alter a human genome through cloning of an embryo awaits no further technical developments. We have already created transgenic plants and animals. A transgenic human is a small scientific, but immense ethical step down a path we have already taken.

Will genetic engineering be used in the treatment and prevention of cancer? Gene therapy, of course, is already in use. Would we ever attempt to correct an inherited loss of a tumor suppressor gene in an embryo destined to have familial adenomatous polyposis? Would we ever wish to transfect routinely all embryos with a gene that confers better resistance to the mutations that cause cancer? Would we wish to change the genetic mechanism that shortens our telomeres, in order to live longer? These questions have no answer today. The fact that the knowledge of the molecular basis of cancer has advanced to the point that we may formulate them is already shocking enough.

Summary

The study of the molecular biology of cancer has resulted in the discovery a large number of target events on which to develop molecular therapies. We can correct, inhibit, or destroy the oncogenes and repair the function of tumor suppressor genes. We can synthesize short pieces of DNA as antisense oligonucleotides to block mRNA from a specific gene. We can transfect engineered gene sequences into tumor cells or cells of the immune system to alter their behavior. We can tranfect bone marrow with genes that render it more resistant to the side effects of conventional chemotherapy. Finally, genetic engineering of humans as a race, in order to make us cancer resistant and possibly longer lived, has become a science fiction idea that is not without technical basis.

References

Askari FK, McDonnell WM. Molecular medicine: antisense-oligonucleotiede therapy. *New Engl J Med.* 1996;334:316–318.

Bischoff JR, Kirn DH, Williams A, et al. An adenovirus mutant that replicates selectively in p53-deficient human tumor cells. *Science.* 1996;274:373–376.

Blaese MR. Gene therapy for cancer. *Sci Am.* 1997;July:111–115.

Current clinical trials in oncology. Physician's data query (PDQ) on-line database, National Cancer Institute. (Also published bimonthly by Pyros Education Group, Green Brook, NJ.)

Ho PTC, Parkinson DR. Antisense oligonucleotides as therapeutics for malignant diseases. *Semin Oncol.* 1997;24:1–17.

Kevles DJ, Hood L, eds. *The Code of Codes: Scientific and Social Issues in the Human Genome Project.* Cambridge: Harvard University Press; 1992.

Conclusions

What have we learned about cancer as a molecular disease? First, cancer is the result of mutations in growth control genes—the oncogenes. Cancer is also a multistep process, of which oncogene mutations are only a part. Mutations must also occur in the genes that protect the cell from DNA damage—the tumor suppressor genes. These mutations disrupt the control of cell proliferation that is built into the genome. The mutated cell passes its abnormalities onto its progeny, establishing a clone of itself. The neoplastic cells, because they have damaged tumor suppressor genes, are genetically unstable. The clone evolves into a tumor that acquires the ability to invade tissues and metastasize.

Molecular lesions always precede, usually by quite some time, the clinical appearance of a tumor. Molecular damage is the basis of carcinogenesis. Chemicals that bind to DNA as adducts or radiation that breaks DNA strands, if unrepaired, starts the process. Our understanding of the molecular biology of cancer leads to diagnostic tests that detect these precursor molecular lesions. In a subset of cancers, inherited germline mutations in tumor suppressor genes such as *BRCA*1 are the causes of genetic predisposition to cancer. We are learning how to use genetic screening to advise affected patients. More commonly, cancer arises from acquired somatic mutations. We are beginning to characterize cancers by their specific molecular lesions. Lymphoma and leukemia are defined more precisely by chromosome translocation and oncogene mutations. The evolution of colon cancer can be staged by the progressive molecular lesions that characterize the evolving neoplasia.

The molecular basis of cancer gives us insight into how cancers may be prevented. Squamous cell carcinoma of the cervix provides an example of molecular damage whose cause is known. Infection with certain strains of human papilloma virus inhibits p53 and *RB*1 tumor suppressor gene function. The infected cells are fertile ground for oncogene mutations that cannot be repaired. HPV vaccines under development will likely cure this disease.

The multiple steps in the evolution of cancer also suggest many new targets for molecular anticancer therapies. We can fix mutated oncogenes and tumor suppressor genes by transfection. We can block specific gene malfunctions through antisense or antibodies. We can destroy cancer cells with genetically engineered viruses. Genetic engineering also allows us to manipulate the immune system to turn it against tumors. We can make tissues such as the bone marrow transgenically resistant to anticancer drugs.

At the beginning of this book, I suggested that you look ahead to Table 11.1, a schematic for new anticancer therapies. Now I recommend that you look back a few pages to that same table. Reflect on what we have learned. Armed with this knowledge of the molecular biology of cancer, we can be hopeful. There is so much more that we know and so much more that we can do.

Glossary

ABL: an oncogene that produces a tyrosine kinase; abnormal expression is seen in chronic myeloid leukemia (CML).

allele: one of possible multiple forms of a gene that can occupy the specific chromosomal location for that gene.

aneuploid: abnormal DNA content (see **diploid**).

angiogenesis: the process of inducing blood supply to new tissues; a factor in allowing tumors to grow.

antioncogene: an outdated term used to describe a **tumor suppressor gene.**

antisense oligonucleotide: a short segment of DNA, synthesized to be complementary in genetic sequence to the sense strand of RNA, used to block gene translation.

APC: a tumor suppressor gene, mutated to loss of function in colon cancer.

apoptosis: (Greek, "fallen leaves") the process whereby a cell commits suicide in response to internal signals.

base pair (bp): the smallest unit of information encoded in DNA, referring to one of the rungs on the double helix of DNA.

***bcl-*2:** an oncogene that inhibits normal cell death via **apoptosis.**

BCR/ABL: a gene fusion that occurs with the **Philadelphia chromosomal translocation**; specific marker for chronic myeloid leukemia.

***BRCA*1:** a tumor suppressor gene that when mutated confers a high risk of hereditary breast and ovary cancer.

carcinogenesis: the study of the multiple steps and causes of neoplastic cell growth.

carcinoma *in situ*: a singular stage in the multistep evolution of cancer in which neoplastic cells are present but without invasion.

cell signaling pathway: a process consisting of a series of proteins, encoded by **proto-oncogenes,** that relays extracellular signals into instructions that affect cell growth.

checkpoint: a point in the cell division cycle where the cell is checked for damage to DNA and held back if damage is found.

chemo-protection: chemicals that protect against chemical carcinogens, such as substances that absorb free radicals.

chromosome: a complex structure of DNA and protein carrying part of the genome, visible under the microscope at cellular mitosis where identical pairs are separated into two daughter cells.

chromosomal translocation: an abnormal process where two chromosomes break and exchange pieces.

clonal: a proliferation of genetically identical cells.

codon: three base pairs along DNA code for a single amino acid during the translation of a gene into protein.

CYCLIN **D1:**   a gene on chromosome 11 that produces a protein involved in cell cycle progression, overexpressed when mutated as an oncogene.

diploid: normal DNA content, or 46 chromosomes and 7 picograms, occurring in most cells; see **aneuploid**.

DNA adduct: a chemical complex binding a carcinogen to DNA.

DNA index: a measure of the amount of DNA in cells, with normal diploid DNA content as a reference index of 1.0—also called ploidy index.

DNA polymerase: an enzyme that enables synthesis of DNA from a DNA template strand.

DNA vaccines: a new class of vaccines based on DNA inserting into the cell; the intracellular translation of this DNA produces MHC type I immunity; a possible vaccination method for HPV and HIV.

dominant: a gene that when present as only one copy out of two alleles produces sufficient functional protein to have an effect; the opposite of **recessive**.

exon: a segment of DNA within a gene that codes for protein, separated from adjacent exons by noncoding segments called **introns**.

familial adenomatous polyposis coli (FAP):   a syndrome due to the inherited loss of the *APC* tumor suppressor gene that results in the development of numerous colon polyps with a high probability of cancer if untreated.

FISH: fluorescent *in situ* hybridization, a method for analysis of chromosomes and DNA by use of fluorescent DNA probes and microscopy.

flow cytometry: the quantitative measure of cellular parameters such as DNA content by laser light scattering technology.

frame shift: a type of mutation in which the reading of triplet **codon** DNA sequences is shifted out of phase producing a **nonsense** message.

G protein: a group of intracytoplasmic proteins coded for by oncogenes; part of the **cell signal pathway**.

G0: a nonproliferating phase of the cell cycle consisting of a reservoir of cells that have completed mitosis but have halted further division.

G1: a phase of the cell division cycle occurring after mitosis (**M**) and before DNA synthesis (**S**).

G2: a phase of the cell division cycle occurring after DNA synthesis (**S**) and before mitosis (**M**).

gene: a segment of DNA that encodes a message, usually the amino acid sequence of a protein as well as information controlling the expression of this information.

genotype: a specific informational set carried as a gene or group of genes, but not necessarily expressed.

germline: the genome of an organism at birth, before any mutations or rearrangements.

graft versus host disease (GVHD): a reaction by transplanted (donor) immune cells against cells of the host.

haploid: half normal DNA content (one half of 46 **chromosomes**) occurring in germ cells; see **diploid**.

her-2/neu: an oncogene coding for a cell surface receptor; overexpressed in 25% to 35% of breast cancers.

hereditary nonpolyposis colon cancer (HNPCC): a syndrome caused by inherited loss of mismatched repair genes.

HPV: human papilloma virus, a factor in viral **carcinogenesis** of squamous cell carcinoma of the cervix.

HSV-tk: a **kit** for transfecting a thymidine kinase gene into a cell using herpes simplex virus as a vector.

HTLV-1: a retrovirus with transforming ability related to adult T-cell lymphoid leukemia.

hybridization: the binding of probe to target, used for DNA and protein molecular studies.

IgH: a symbol for the immunoglobulin heavy chain gene.

image cytometry: the quantitative measure of cellular parameters by computer assisted microscopy.

initiator: a chemical carcinogen that is part of the process of inducing mutations that cause neoplastic proliferation.

intron: a segment of DNA within a gene that does not code for a protein, occurring as a space between **exons.**

in vitro: (Latin, "in glass") a process studied outside the body, usually in a cell culture.

karyotype: an analysis of the chromosome content of cells by microscopic examination. A normal human karyotype is 46XY or 46XX.

kit: a commercially available packaged process consisting of the methods and materials necessary to carry out a fundament step in biotechnology.

loss of heterozygosity (LOH):   a genetic mechanism that results in damage to the second allele of a gene by incorrect copying or conversion from the first mutated allele.

M: mitosis, a phase of the cell division cycle, recognizable by the appearance of **chromosomes.**

MDR: multi-drug resistance gene; produces a 170-kd glycoprotein that pumps toxic substances out of a cell; amplification of this gene is a mechanism for drug resistance in tumors.

microsatellite instability: a genetic phenomenon in which short repeating DNA sequences undergo multiple and varying repeats when copied; leads to further mutations.

mismatch repair genes: a group of DNA repair genes, also classified as tumor suppressor genes that when mutated lead to **microsatellite instability** and further mutation, a cause of **HNPCC** syndrome.

mutation: a change in DNA that produces a change in phenotype, usually away from what is considered to be normal (see **polymorphism**).

myc: a family of oncogenes that produce a DNA transcription factor that stimulates cell division.

neoplastic: a cellular proliferation not under normal controls; may be clinically benign or malignant.

neural network: a computational method that allows for comparison of multiple parameters affecting a process.

nonsense: a DNA segment that does not code for amino acids having no open reading frame.

Northern blot: a method of analyzing RNA.

oncogene: the mutated form of a growth control gene; a step in the formation of a tumor.

open reading frame, ORF: a long segment of DNA that when read as triplets, produces a set of codons that does not include a STOP codon; an ORF is a sign that this segment of DNA is part of a gene.

p53: a **tumor suppressor gene** mutated in many cancers resulting in loss of a **checkpoint** for DNA damage.

PCR: polymerase chain reaction, a method for amplifying pieces of DNA; used as a detection method and to produce pieces for further study; a mainstay of recombinant DNA technology.

pharming: the process of creating new molecules by growing them in genetically altered plants or animals.

Philadelphia chromosome: a **t(9;22) chromosomal translocation** that is a marker for the neoplastic clone in chronic myeloid leukemia.

phenotype: the physical expression of a specific gene or group of genes; see **genotype**.

polymorphism: a change in DNA that produces no change in phenotype.

promoter: a substance that stimulates cell growth such that when combined with a chemical **initiator** leads to neoplastic cell growth, part of **carcinogenesis**.

proto-oncogene: the normal cellular form of a gene that controls cell growth, that when mutated becomes an **oncogene**.

recessive: a gene that only when present as both copies of two possible alleles results in a characteristic phenotype; the opposite of **dominant**.

replicon: a structure on the DNA strand that carries out the functions of copying during DNA synthesis.

restriction enzyme: an enzyme, derived from bacteria that cuts DNA at a specific site based on nucleotide sequence; a major tool of recombinant DNA technology.

retrovirus: an RNA virus that uses the cell's own genes to help it replicate; posesses the unique enzyme **reverse transcriptase**.

reverse transcriptase: an enzyme that copies RNA into DNA, reversing the normal flow of genetic information.

S: a phase of the cell division cycle in which DNA synthesis occurs.

S phase fraction: the percent of cells in a tissue that are currently synthesizing DNA; a measure by **cytometry** of the cell proliferation.

somatic (line): refers to the genome of tissues that may be altered from the **germline** by mutation or rearrangement.

Southern blot: a method for analyzing DNA by electrophoresis and hybridization blotting, named after Ed Southern.

splice acceptor site: a DNA sequence where DNA is cut and re-arranged; these sites seem predisposed to erroneous rejoining and **chromosomal translocation**.

src: a **viral oncogene** with **transforming** ability seen in the Rous sarcoma retrovirus.

t(9;22): karyotype nomenclature for the **Philadelphia chromosome** and *BCR/ABL* gene fusion seen in chronic myeloid leukemia.

Taq: a special **DNA polymerase** that is stable at high temperatures; used in PCR; pronounced "tack."

telomerase: a DNA polymerase that replicates **telomeres**; may be abnormal in tumor cells allowing unlimited numbers of cell division.

telomere: a genetic element at the end of a chromosome consisting of a repetitive DNA sequence that becomes progressively shorter with each cell division.

tetraploid: twice normal DNA content, or 92 chromosomes occurring in dividing cells just before mitosis, also occurring abnormally in some tumors.

transform: a genetic mutation that results in continuous cell growth **in vitro**.

transgenic: an organism whose heredity has been altered by biotechnology.

viral oncogene: the viral form of a cell growth control gene or **proto-oncogene**, seen in some **retroviruses.**

Western blot: a method for analyzing proteins.

185delAG: a specific deletion in the *BRCA1* breast cancer susceptibility gene; refers to a deletion of nucleotides A and G at position 185 in the gene.

Index